ISBN: 9781070491202

Note: At publication, the off-the-shelf foods used in this book were widely available in most supermarkets. But food products come and go. So if there is a frozen entrée or soup selection in this diet that is out of stock, or that's been discontinued, or perhaps you don't like, or that you forgot to pick up while shopping, please substitute another food that has **approximately** the same caloric value and nutritional content. In this regard, many dieters have found the foods listed in the Appendices at the end of this book to be very helpful.

30-DAY
VEGETARIAN DIET
PESCETARIAN

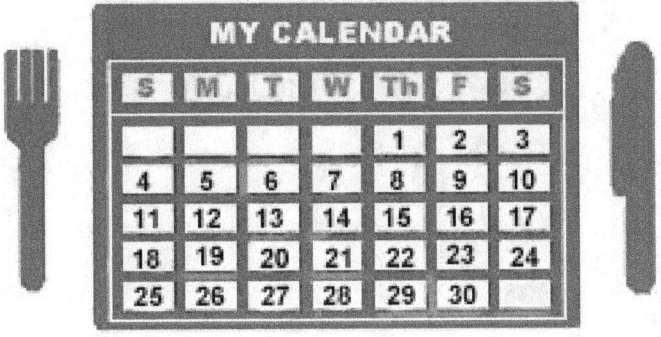

S. Vjay Gupta

Gail Johnson, M.S.

NoPaperPress™

CONTENTS

The 30-Day Vegetarian Diet blends American cooking with Asian vegetarian concepts. Of course this diet is meatless, but fish, eggs and dairy are allowed. The diet is a Pescetarian version of vegetarianism and features delicious, low calorie, nutritionally balanced vegetarian meals.

A well planned vegetarian diet can provide the same level of nutrients as a meat-eater's diet. In addition, eating meat-free can have real weight-loss benefits because plant-based foods, such as vegetables, beans and whole grains, are loaded with fiber that help you feel satisfied on fewer calories. And many health-care professionals also think that eating a healthy vegetarian diet is one of the best things you can do for your short-term and long-term health.

Vegetarian Types

When deciding what type of vegetarian you want to be, think about what foods you want to include or avoid. There are several vegetarian versions:

1. **Lacto-Ovo Vegetarians** do not eat animal flesh of any kind (including beef, pork, poultry, fish and shellfish) but they do eat eggs and dairy products. This is the most popular vegetarian diet.

2. **Lacto-Vegetarians** do not eat animal flesh of any kind (including beef, pork, poultry, fish and shellfish) and do not eat meat or eggs – but do consume dairy products.

3. **Ovo-Vegetarians** do not eat animal flesh of any kind (including beef, pork, poultry, fish and shellfish) and do not eat meat or dairy products – but do eat eggs.

4. **Pesceterians** do not eat meat or poultry but do eat eggs, dairy and fish. Some Pesceterians also eat other seafood (shrimp, scallops, etc.). People often adopt this diet for health reasons, or as a stepping stone to a fully vegetarian diet. This vegetarian version is sometimes called Semi-Vegetarian.

5. **Vegans** are strict vegetarians who do not eat meat of any kind and also do not eat eggs, dairy products, or processed foods containing these or other animal-derived ingredients. Many vegans also refrain from eating foods that are made using animal products even though the food may not contain animal products in the finished product, such as sugar and some wines.

With this eBook, NoPaperPress publishes a popular vegetarian variant: the **Pesceterian Vegetarian Diet** that includes fish, eggs and dairy products. And all NoPaperPress vegetarian diet eBooks come in 90-day, 30-day and 7-day editions. For background and nutritional information and more on vegetarianism see **Appendix A** (page 111).

The Best Weight-Loss Diets

According to the late Dr. Jean Mayer of Harvard University's Department of Nutrition, a really good weight-loss diet must have the following three characteristics:

1) The diet must provide you with an understanding of weight control as well as the knowledge you need to reduce your weight to the desired level.

2) The diet must help you remain healthy while you are losing weight.

3) The diet must lead you to a healthier way of eating and exercising that will, in the long term, help you keep off the weight you have lost.

The weight-loss diet featured in this eBook is a "balanced diet;" i.e., a diet that is not only low calorie and reasonably low in fat, but is also nutritionally balanced. The *30-Day Vegetarian Diet*, however, does not meet all the criteria set forth above. While you will get some "dieting insight" and some idea of how much you can eat and still lose weight, you will not get a real understanding of weight control from this eBook. That's not its purpose. What you will get is a healthy diet – and a diet that if followed will promote weight loss. Think of the *30-Day Vegetarian Diet* as a quick fix, a healthy start that will get you on the right track – but it's not the long-term answer.

Long-term success is about developing both an understanding and a plan that will result in healthier eating and physical activity habits. For a through understanding and the guidance you need to succeed in the long term I recommend you read, *Weight Control - U.S. Edition* by Vincent Antonetti, Ph.D., a NoPaperPress eBook

Begin with a Medical Exam

Everyone should at the very least have a medical assessment, or exam, before starting a weight loss diet. Why? You need to make sure your health will allow you to lower your caloric intake and increase your physical activity. The medical checkup may be as simple as a visit to a physician who is familiar with your medical history, or it may be a thorough physical exam. The physician conducting the medical exam should be made aware of and should approve the specific weight loss diet you're planning.

What's in This eBook?

This eBook actually contains two 30-day diets: a 1500 Calorie diet, and for even faster weight loss a 1200 Calorie diet. And both diets have a meal plan (menu) for each and every one of the 30 days.

Which Calorie Level is for You?

1200 Calorie Vegetarian Diet: Smaller women, older women and inactive women should select the 1200 Calorie diet.

1500 Calorie Vegetarian Diet: Larger women, younger women and active women and <u>most men</u> should choose the 1500 Calorie diet.

Expected Weight Loss

Weight loss occurs when your food energy intake is less than the total energy you expend. This difference in calories is referred to as your <u>calorie deficit</u>. How much weight you lose depends on the magnitude of your calorie deficit. Simple metabolic calculations make a rough estimate possible.

On the 30-Day Vegetarian Diet, <u>**most women lose 10 to 15 pounds**</u> – depending on whether the 1500 or 1200 Calorie diet is selected. Smaller women, older women and less active women will lose a bit less and larger women, younger women and more active women often more.

On the 30-Day Vegetarian Diet, <u>**most men lose 15 to 20 pounds**</u> – depending on whether the 1500 or 1200 Calorie diet is selected. Smaller men, older men and less active men will lose a bit less and larger men, younger men and more active men often much more. Exactly how much weight you will lose depends on how much you weigh, your age and your activity level. Again, for the full story see *Weight Control - U.S. Edition* by Vincent Antonetti, Ph.D.

Guidelines for Healthy Eating

No single food can supply all the nutrients you need in the amounts you need. The most important factors in nutrition are variety, variety, variety! **Variety is the key to a nutritious diet.** As a means of setting strategies for food selection, the U.S. Department of Health and Human Services and the Department of Agriculture issue Dietary Guidelines every five years. The latest Dietary Guidelines describe a healthy diet as one that:

- Emphasizes fruits, vegetables, whole grains, and fat-free or low-fat milk

products.
- Includes fish, beans and nuts.
- Is low in saturated fats, trans fats, cholesterol, salt (sodium) and added sugars.

The guidelines encourage adults to consume a variety of nutrient-dense foods and beverages within their caloric needs. The afore mentioned U.S. government agency recommends how much should be eaten from each of the basic food groups (i.e., from the fruit group, vegetable group, grains group, beans group, milk group, and oils group) – whether you are trying to lose weight or maintain your weight. All this information and more can be found in my eBook *Eat Smart - U.S. Edition* published by NoPaperPress.

Even though most adults can get all the vitamins and minerals they need by merely consuming a variety of nutritious foods (from the fruit group, the vegetable group, the grains group, the meat and beans group, the milk group, and the oils group), many physicians recommend a daily multi-vitamin/mineral supplement – just in case you don't eat the way you should.

Large Green Salad: One of the dinner mainstays is a "Large Green Salad." Prepare your "Large Green Salad" in a bowl with a volume of at least 16 ounces, or 2 cups. First add about 1 cup of either green leaf lettuce, Romaine lettuce or a mesclun mix. Then add, as desired, half cup of green veggies such as broccoli, celery, cucumber, peppers, spinach, or watercress. This vegetable combination will, on average, total about 35 Calories. You will be eating a "Large Green Salad" just about every day at dinnertime. Remember that variety is the key to a nutritious diet. So be sure to vary the ingredients of the salad.

Top your "Large Green Salad" with 1½ tablespoons of any light salad dressing available at your local supermarket that contains no more than 25 Calories per tablespoon. Some of our favorite light salad dressings are:
  - **Kraft Light Done Right House Italian**
  - **Wishbone Just 2 Good Honey Dijon**
  - **Newman's Lighten Up! Balsamic Vinaigrette**
Your "Large Green Salad" with salad dressing will cost you roughly 70 Calories but will be packed with lots of health-giving vitamins, minerals and fiber. (Remember to check the labels of all processed products to assure that they are vegetarian.)

About Bread: First understand that bread, more specifically whole-grain breads, are good sources of complex carbohydrates and dietary fiber, as well as several B vitamins (thiamin, riboflavin, niacin, and foliate), vitamin E, and minerals (iron, magnesium and selenium). In recent years, however, sliced bread loaves have gotten larger, as have the bread slices inside these loaves. Just a few years ago the standard slice of bread contained about 65 to 70 Calories – now most are 100 plus Calories.

The *30-Day Vegetarian Diet* **requires whole-grain bread at 65 to 70 Calories per slice.** Quite a few bakers sell thin sliced or "light" sliced bread. The difficult part is finding a whole grain thin sliced or "light" bread (with about 70 Calories per slice). Whatever the brand, make sure the first word in the Ingredients list is "whole." "Pepperidge Farm Small Slice 100% Whole Wheat" is a good choice. It's whole grain, has 70 Calories per slice and it tastes good too.

Exchanging Foods

If there is a food listed in the *30-Day Vegetarian Diet* that you don't like, or perhaps that you forgot to pick up while shopping, you probably can exchange or substitute another food in its place – a technique used by dieticians. Exchanging a food listed in a diet for another food with approximately equal caloric value and nutritional content is the foundation of a successful long-term diet. Substitution possibilities are almost endless but have to be done carefully.

The easiest substitutions are those within the same food group, such as exchanging one vegetable variety for another, or a glass of milk for a cup of yogurt. More sophisticated exchanges cross food groups, for instance replacing 3½ ounces of turkey with a tablespoon of peanut butter spread on a piece of whole grain bread. Both foods are complete protein and both contain about 175 Calories.

Refer to the calorie table in **Appendix D** (page 120) . With some understanding and experience, you can use this table to help you substitute foods called for in the *30-Day Vegetarian Diet* with equal calorie foods from the same food group.

Breakfast: You may substitute any cereal for any other wholesome cereal. For example, if you're not crazy about having Shredded Wheat for breakfast on Day 6, substitute Wheat Chex or Cheerios, etc. If you don't like the soft-boiled egg called for on Day 9, make yourself a scrambled egg instead. And if Cantaloupe is on the menu but is not in season, replace the cantaloupe with a half cup of orange juice.

Snacks: Again, where yogurt is specified you may substitute an 8-ounce glass of skim milk, but to maintain a nutritionally balanced diet keep this snack a dairy selection. Similarly, when fruit is on the agenda, you may select another type of fruit but do not stray from the fruit group. Nuts and popcorn can be interchanged at will. (Incidentally, you should buy a hot-air popper. They make great popcorn – which is high in fiber and makes a tasty and nutritious snack.)

Two Nights Off

Everyone deserves a break from the grind of preparing dinner after coming home from work. So the *30-Day Vegetarian Diet* gives you two days off per week! Notice that one night a week the meal plan calls for a frozen dinner and on a second night during the week you're encouraged to eat out. There are, however, some rules and caveats involved and these are covered in the next two sections.

Frozen Dinners

In general, a frozen dinner should not be a meal in itself. Make sure you add a salad, fruit, bread etc. The frozen dinner you choose should come with at least one cup of cooked vegetables. If your frozen dinner doesn't measure up, add your own frozen, fresh or canned vegetables. And look for dinners with no more than 800 mg of sodium. In addition, make sure the dinner you choose has no more than 30 percent of the daily value for total fat. Some reasonably good frozen dinner choices are:
  – **Amy's: Asian Noodle Stir-Fry** (300 Calories)
  – **Amy's: Indian Vegetable Korma** (310 Calories)
  – **Amy's: Tofu Scramble** (320 Calories)
  – **Lean Cuisine: Shrimp Alfredo** (200 Calories)
  – **Smart Ones: Pasta Primavera** (250 Calories)

And on the days when a frozen dinner is specified, you will also be given a calorie goal for the frozen dinner. For example, Day 5 calls for frozen fish dinner with a maximum allowable 340 Calories. If you choose a frozen fish dinner that contains less than 340 Calories, you may spend the unused calories any way you wish.

Moreover, on those nights when you just don't have the energy or time to cook, you can always substitute a frozen dinner for the entree listed in the meal plan. For example, Day 1 calls for Herb-Crusted Cod for dinner. The total calorie count for dinner is 530. In place of the cod, any combination of a frozen fish dinner and side dishes (salads, etc) with a total calorie content close to 530 would be an acceptable, albeit not as tasty, alternative.

Eating Out

On this diet, you are encouraged to eat out once a week. When you're on a diet, however, eating in a restaurant can be a challenge, even in a vegetarian establishment, because most restaurant portions are huge, and can easily total more than 1,000 Calories. On the *90-Day Vegetarian Diet*, a dinner type (i.e., fish, tofu, pasta, etc) and a calorie target are specified. For example Day 7 of the 1,500 Calorie diet calls for dinner in a vegetarian restaurant and allows you 630 Calories.

First, you need to choose a restaurant where you have a fighting chance to achieve your calorie goal. Next, order something simple, such as stir-fried tofu with steamed vegetables and brown rice. Tell the waiter you want no sauce, no gravy, nothing added. Then, knowing your calorie objective, and that most stir-fried tofu have less than 35 Calories per ounce, most steamed vegetable servings average approximately 50 Calories per cup, and rice is about 100 Calories per ½ cup, decide how much to eat – and take the remainder home. If fresh fruit is not an option, pass on dessert and have the evening snack specified in the *90-Day Vegetarian Diet* meal plan for that day.

On the days a fish dinner is specified, order broiled fish, and note that most broiled fish are about 50 Calories per ounce. On days when pasta is specified, always order pasta with a marinara sauce or pasta primavera. Generally pasta is 45 Calories per ounce and marinara sauce about 70 Calories per ½ cup.

When you eat out, we recommend you use a calculator app on your smart phone to add up the calories in your meal. And keep a file on your phone with the approximate Calories per ounce of the food you are likely to eat when dinning at a restaurant.

30-Day Diet Info

As mentioned previously, there are two diet plans in this eBook:
  - 1500 Calorie 30-Day Diet starts on page 14.
  - 1200 Calorie 30-Day Diet starts on page 45.
Both have a detailed meal plan for each of the 30 days. Associated with each day is a "recipe of the day" and with most of the days a "Diet Tip of the Day."

The 1200 and 1500 Calorie diets adhere to the United States Department of Agriculture recommendation that suggest a balanced diet should have approximately 50 percent of its calories from carbs, about 20 percent from protein sources and 30 percent or less from fat. (Note, the *30-Day Vegetarian Diet* may not be appropriate for individuals with illnesses such as heart disease, diabetes, food allergies, etc. Again, please see your physician before starting this diet – or any diet.)

After you complete the 30th day on the diet, if you still want to lose more weight a good alternative is to repeat the diet by starting over at Day 1.

Important Notes

1) If desired, skim milk and a sugar substitute may be added to coffee or tea. Coffee or tea may be decaf or regular.

2) Fried or scrambled eggs should be cooked in a pan coated with a non-stick cooking spray. Hard-boiled eggs may be substituted for fried, scrambled or soft-boiled eggs.

3) Cereals should be whole grain and unsweetened. At the top of the list are Old-fashioned Oatmeal, Wheatena and Shredded Wheat. Among other reasonably healthy choices are Cheerios, Wheat Chex, Wheaties, some Kashi cereals and Farina. When blueberries are in season, you may add **blueberries instead of raisins** to your cereal. (Substitution ratio = 2 blueberries per raisin.)

4) Bread may be either plain or toasted, but should be whole grain. Look for whole grain varieties that contain 70 Calories per slice. If desired, bread may be sprayed with a zero-calorie butter substitute. BUT NO BUTTER!

5) When canned soup or in a microwaveable bowl is specified, eat only one serving (8 ounces) unless otherwise noted. (Soup cans and microwaveable bowls usually contain about two servings.)

6) Use freely as desired: clear unsweetened coffee, clear unsweetened tea, water, seltzer water and any diet soda, clear soups without fat, bouillon, and seasonings such as mustard, cinnamon, dill, herbs, red and black pepper, curry, vinegar, lemon juice and sections, and dill and sour pickles.

7) When canned tuna or salmon is specified, use only fish packed in water.

8) An unlimited amount of green salad may be eaten, but the salad dressing should be as specified.

9) If it's more convenient, any food item may be moved to any part of the day and combined with any meal or snack.

10) If you cannot find the exact item called for in the diet (because it's out of stock or discontinued), substitute a comparable food (of the same type and close caloric value).

11) Although it's recommended that you follow the diet days as specified, it's fine to occasionally skip a day and/or pick and choose the days you prefer. (Nutritionally, each day stands on its own.)

12) Finally, NoPaperPress works hard to keep the information in our eBooks up to date. But we recommend that you check the labels of all processed products in this diet to assure that they are still truly vegetarian and that the caloric content is as noted in this book.

1500-Calorie Daily Menus

Day 1 – 1500 Calorie Plan

BREAKFAST	Calories	Totals
Orange juice (½ cup)	50	
Wheaties (¾ cup) + ½ cup skim milk + ½ banana	190	
Whole-grain toast (1 slice) (See page 9)	70	
Coffee (page 12)	10	320 Cal
SNACK		
Fresh fruit in season (apple, pear, etc)	70	
Coffee or tea	10	80 Cal
LUNCH		
Soup (Appendix B - page 116)	60	
Sliced hard-boiled egg on 2 slices bread	230	
Lettuce & tomato slices	20	
Hot or iced tea	10	320 Cal
SNACK		
Popcorn Mini Bag*	110	
Coffee or tea	10	120 Cal
DINNER		
Baked Herb-Crusted Cod (Day 1 Recipe - page 77)	230	
Spinach (½ cup) steamed with garlic & drizzled	100	
Asparagus (8 spears cooked & drained)	25	
Baked potato (medium size) (No Butter!)	100	
Whole-grain bread (1 slice)	70	
Water	0	525 Cal
SNACK		
Skinny Cow Ice Cream Sandwich	140	140 Cal
* Such as Orville Redenbacher's Smart Pop		1505 Cal

Day 2 – 1500 Calorie Plan

BREAKFAST	Calories	Totals
Fresh or frozen strawberries (½ cup)	25	
French-toasted English Muffin Day 2a Recipe - page 78)	270	
Light syrup (1 Tbsp)	30	
Coffee	10	335 Cal
SNACK		
Yogurt (6 oz, nonfat, any flavor)*	90	
Coffee or tea	10	100 Cal
LUNCH		
Salad (3 oz tuna, 1 tsp Evoo, onions & celery)	175	
Lettuce & tomato wedges	20	
Rye bread (1 slice)	65	
Fresh fruit in season (apple, plum, etc)	70	
Coffee or tea	10	340 Cal
SNACK		
Handful unsalted mixed nuts	100	
Coffee or tea	10	110 Cal
DINNER		
Polenta-stuffed peppers (Day 2b Recipe -page 79)	290	
Large green salad with 1½ Tbsp low-cal dressing	70	
Small whole-grain roll	80	
Water with lemon wedge	10	450 Cal
SNACK		
Skinny Cow Ice Cream Sandwich	140	
Coffee or tea	10	150 Cal
* Such as Dannon Lite & Fit. (Buy 32 oz container & use 6 oz.)		1490 Cal

Day 3 – 1500 Calorie Meal Plan

BREAKFAST	Calories	Totals
Orange juice (½ cup)	50	
Scrambled egg (page 12)	80	
Whole-grain toast (2 slices)	140	
Coffee	10	280 Cal
SNACK		
Handful unsalted mixed nuts	100	
Coffee or tea	10	110 Cal
LUNCH		
Peanut butter (1 Tbsp) on 1 slice whole-grain bread	170	
Skim milk (6 oz)	70	
Fresh fruit in season (apple, peach, etc)	70	
Hot or iced tea	10	320 Cal
SNACK		
Kashi TLC Chewy Granola Bar	140	140 Cal
DINNER		
Crumbly-Tofu Scramble (Day 3 Recipe - page 80)	240	
Four small white potatoes - roasted	210	
Large green salad + 1½ Tbsp low-cal dressing (page 8)	70	
Water with lemon section	10	530 Cal
SNACK		
Graham crackers (4 squares)	120	
Coffee or tea	10	130 Cal
		1510 Cal

Day 4 – 1500 Calorie Meal Plan

BREAKFAST	Calories	Totals
Grapefruit (½)	75	
Cheerios (1 cup) + ½ cup skim milk + about 15 raisins*	190	
Coffee	10	275 Cal
SNACK		
Fresh fruit in season (apple, peach, etc)	70	
Coffee or tea	10	80 Cal
LUNCH		
Cottage cheese (1 cup low fat)	180	
Large green salad with 2 Tbsp low-cal dressing	85	
Small whole-grain roll	80	
Water	0	345 Cal
SNACK		
Handful unsalted mixed nuts	100	100 Cal
DINNER		
Easy Penne Pasta (Day 4 Recipe - page 81)	375	
Italian or French bread (1 slice)	80	
Glass red wine (4 oz)	100	
Water	0	555 Cal
SNACK		
Skinny Cow Ice Cream Sandwich	140	
Coffee or tea	10	150 Cal
* See page 12 re substituting blueberries for raisins.		1505 Cal

Day 5 – 1500 Calorie Meal Plan

BREAKFAST	Calories	Totals
Cantaloupe (½ medium)	50	
Fried egg	80	
Toasted raisin bread (1 slice)	75	
Coffee	10	215 Cal
SNACK		
Yogurt (6 oz, nonfat, any flavor)	90	
Coffee or tea	10	100 Cal
LUNCH		
Soup (Appendix B - page 116)	140	
Small whole-grain roll	80	
Lettuce and sliced tomato with 1 Tbsp low-cal	45	
Canned pineapple (½ cup, no-sugar-added juice)	40	
Hot or iced tea	10	315 Cal
SNACK		
Popcorn Mini Bag	110	
Coffee or tea	10	120 Cal
DINNER		
Frozen fish dinner (Day 5 Recipe - page 82)	340	
Large green salad with 1½ Tbsp low-cal dressing	70	
Small whole-grain roll	80	
Fresh fruit in season (apple, peach, etc)	70	
Water with lemon wedge	10	570 Cal
SNACK		
Dark chocolate (1 oz)	150	
Coffee or tea	10	160 Cal
		1480 Cal

Day 6 – 1500 Calorie Meal Plan

BREAKFAST	Calories	Totals
Tomato juice (½ cup)	20	
Shredded Wheat (1 cup) + ½ cup skim milk + ½ banana	265	
Coffee	10	295 Cal
SNACK		
Handful unsalted mixed nuts	100	
Coffee or tea	10	110 Cal
LUNCH		
Salad – 3 oz canned salmon + 1 tsp Evoo, onions & celery	200	
Small whole-grain roll	80	
Lettuce	0	
Hot or iced tea	10	290 Cal
SNACK		
Yogurt (6 oz, nonfat, any flavor)	90	
Coffee or tea	10	100 Cal
DINNER		
Pizza (Day 6 Recipe - page 83)	350	
Large green salad with 1½ Tbsp low-cal dressing	70	
Fresh fruit in season (peach, plum, etc)	70	
Glass of red wine (4 oz)	100	
Water with lemon section	10	600 Cal
SNACK		
100-Calorie Pack Cookies*	100	
Coffee or tea	10	110 Cal
* Such as Nabisco Oreo/Chips Ahoy/etc		1505 Cal

Day 7 – 1500 Calorie Meal Plan

BREAKFAST	Calories	Totals
Cantaloupe (½ medium)	50	
Oatmeal (½ cup dry) + ½ cup skim milk + about 15 raisins	220	
Coffee	10	280 Cal
SNACK		
Fresh fruit in season (pear, plum, etc)	70	
Coffee or tea	10	80 Cal
LUNCH		
Soup (Appendix B - page 116)	100	
Grilled cheese sandwich (2 slices 2% American	230	
Lettuce and sliced tomato	20	
Pickle spear	0	
Water	0	350 Cal
SNACK		
Carrot sticks + ¼ cup low-fat cottage cheese & chives	60	
Coffee or tea	10	70 Cal
DINNER		
Eat Out - Vegetarian dinner (Day 7 Recipe - page 84)		
Max allowable calories	630	630 Cal
SNACK		
Graham crackers (3 squares)	90	
Coffee or tea	10	100 Cal
		1510 Cal

Day 8 – 1500 Calorie Meal Plan

BREAKFAST	Calories	Totals
Cantaloupe (½ medium)	50	
Wheaties (¾ cup) + ½ cup skim milk + ½ banana	190	
Whole-grain toast (1 slice)	70	
Coffee	10	320 Cal
SNACK		
Handful unsalted mixed nuts	100	
Coffee or tea	10	110 Cal
LUNCH		
Soup (Appendix B - page 116)	150	
Lettuce & tomato sandwich (plus Tbsp light mayo)	150	
Fresh fruit in season (peach, plum, etc)	70	
Hot or iced tea	10	380 Cal
SNACK		
Popcorn Mini Bag	110	
Coffee or tea	10	120 Cal
DINNER		
Baked salmon with salsa (Day 8 Recipe - page 85)	215	
Summer squash and zucchini	40	
Medium tomato - sliced	20	
Brown rice (½ cup – after cooking)	100	
Large green salad with 1½ Tbsp low-cal dressing	70	
Water with lemon wedge	10	455 Cal
SNACK		
Graham crackers (2 squares)	60	
Skim milk (4 oz)	45	105 Cal
		1490 Cal

Day 9 – 1500 Calorie Meal Plan

BREAKFAST	Calories	Totals
Fresh orange sliced	75	
Kashi GoLean (1 cup) + ½ cup skim milk + ½ banana	235	
Whole-grain toast (1 slice)	70	
Coffee	10	390 Cal
SNACK		
Fresh fruit in season (apple, plum, etc)	70	
Coffee or tea	10	80 Cal
LUNCH		
Soup (Appendix B - page 116)	140	
Small whole-grain roll	80	
Raw zucchini slices, celery and carrot sticks	20	
Hot or iced tea	10	250 Cal
SNACK		
Popcorn Mini Bag	110	
Coffee or tea	10	120 Cal
DINNER		
Portobello mushroom burger (Day 9 Recipe -page 86)	270	
Lettuce and sliced tomato	20	
Whole-grain hard roll	140	
Steamed green beans	25	
Pickle spear	0	
Water with lemon wedge	10	465 Cal
SNACK		
Two small cookies*	160	
Skim milk (4 oz)	45	205 Cal
*Sugar cookie, chocolate chip, etc - check calories!		1510 Cal

Day 10 – 1500 Calorie Meal Plan

BREAKFAST	Calories	Totals
Orange juice (½ cup)	50	
Wild blueberry pancakes (Day 10 Recipe - page 87)	190	
Light syrup (1½ Tbsp)	45	
Coffee	10	365 Cal
SNACK		
Yogurt (6 oz, nonfat, any flavor)	90	
Coffee or tea	10	100 Cal
LUNCH		
Péanut butter (2 Tbsp) on 2 slices whole-grain bread	330	
Skim milk (6 oz)	65	
Fresh fruit in season (apple, peach, etc)	70	465 Cal
SNACK		
Carrot sticks + ¼ cup low-fat cottage cheese & chives	60	
Coffee or tea	10	70 Cal
DINNER		
Eggplant Parmesan (Day 10b Recipe - page 88)	270	
Large green salad with 1½ Tbsp low-cal dressing	70	
Italian or French bread (1 slice)	80	
Water	0	430 Cal
SNACK		
Graham crackers (2 squares)	60	
Coffee or tea	10	70 Cal
		1500 Cal

Day 11 – 1500 Calorie Meal Plan

BREAKFAST	Calories	Totals
Fresh sliced orange	75	
Cheerios (1 cup) + ½ cup skim milk + about 15 raisins	240	
Whole-grain toast (1 slice)	70	
Coffee	10	395 Cal
SNACK		
Popcorn Mini Bag	110	
Coffee or tea	10	120 Cal
LUNCH		
Cottage cheese (1 cup low fat)	180	
Large green salad with 1½ Tbsp low-cal dressing	70	
Small whole-grain roll	80	
Hot or iced tea	10	340 Cal
SNACK		
Handful unsalted mixed nuts	100	
Coffee or tea	10	110 Cal
DINNER		
Mexican Beans and Rice (Day 11 Recipe - page 89)	270	
Whole-grain bread (1 slice)	70	
Fresh fruit in season (peach, plum, etc)	70	
Water with lemon wedge	10	420 Cal
SNACK		
100-Calorie Pack Cookies	100	
Coffee or tea	10	110 Cal
		1495 Cal

Day 12 – 1500 Calorie Meal Plan

BREAKFAST	Calories	Totals
Grapefruit (½)	75	
Scrambled egg	80	
Whole-grain toast (2 slices)	140	
Coffee	10	305 Cal
SNACK		
Yogurt (6 oz, nonfat, any flavor)	90	
Coffee or tea	10	100 Cal
LUNCH		
Soup (Appendix B - page 116)	160	
Tomato slices w ¼ cup chopped fresh basil + 1 tsp Evoo	60	
Whole-grain bread (1 slice)	65	
Gelatin dessert (unsweetened)	10	
Hot or iced tea	10	305 Cal
SNACK		
Fresh fruit in season (apple, plum, etc)	70	
Coffee or tea	10	80 Cal
DINNER		
Eat Out – Fish dinner (Day 12 Recipe - page 90)		
Max allowable calories	595	595 Cal
SNACK		
Graham crackers (4 squares)	120	
Coffee or tea	10	130 Cal
		1515 Cal

Day 13 – 1500 Calorie Meal Plan

BREAKFAST	Calories	Totals
Orange juice (½ cup)	50	
Shredded Wheat (1 cup) + ½ cup skim milk + ½ banana	260	
Whole-grain toast (1 slice)	70	
Coffee	10	390 Cal
SNACK		
Handful unsalted mixed nuts	100	
Coffee or tea	10	110 Cal
LUNCH		
Egg salad (1 egg + 1 Tbsp light mayo)	125	
Small whole-grain roll	80	
Lettuce and sliced tomato with 1 Tbsp low-cal	45	
Hot or iced tea	10	260 Cal
SNACK		
Kashi TLC Chewy Granola Bar	140	
Coffee or tea	10	150 Cal
DINNER		
Pasta with Marinara sauce (Day 13 Recipe - page 91)	225	
Large green salad with 1½ Tbsp low-cal dressing	70	
Fresh fruit in season (apple, plum, etc)	70	
Italian or French bread (1 slice)	80	
Water	0	445 Cal
SNACK		
Skinny Cow Ice Cream Sandwich	140	
Coffee or tea	10	150 Cal
		1505 Cal

Day 14 – 1500 Calorie Meal Plan

BREAKFAST	Calories	Totals
Cantaloupe (½ medium)	50	
Low-Cal Smoothie (Day 14a Recipe - page 92)	220	
Coffee	10	280 Cal
SNACK		
Handful unsalted mixed nuts	100	100 Cal
LUNCH		
Grilled Swiss cheese sandwich (2 oz low-fat cheese)	310	
Pickle spear	0	
Hot or iced tea	10	330 Cal
SNACK		
Popcorn Mini Bag	110	
Coffee or tea	10	120 Cal
DINNER		
Frozen Fish dinner (Day 14b Recipe - page 93)	300	
Large green salad with 1½ Tbsp low-cal dressing	70	
Whole-grain bread (1 slice)	70	
Fresh fruit in season (apple, peach, etc)	70	
Water	0	510 Cal
SNACK		
Dark chocolate (1 oz)	150	
Coffee or tea	10	160 Cal
		1505 Cal

Day 15 – 1500 Calorie Meal Plan

BREAKFAST	Calories	Totals
Grapefruit (½)	75	
French toast (made w 2 slices whole-grain bread)	250	
Light syrup (1 Tbsp)	30	
Coffee	10	365 Cal
SNACK		
Yogurt (6 oz, nonfat, any flavor)	90	
Coffee or tea	10	100 Cal
LUNCH		
Tuna salad (3 oz tuna, 1 tsp Evoo, onions & celery)	175	
Lettuce & tomato wedges	20	
Rye bread (1 slice)	70	
Coffee or tea	10	275 Cal
SNACK		
Popcorn Mini Bag	110	
Coffee or tea	10	120 Cal
DINNER		
Veggies with Couscous (Day 15 Recipe - page 94)	320	
Small whole-grain roll	80	
Fresh fruit in season (pear, plum, etc)	70	
Water with lemon wedge	10	490 Cal
SNACK		
Graham crackers (4 squares)	120	
Coffee or tea	10	130 Cal
		1480 Cal

Day 16 – 1500 Calorie Meal Plan

BREAKFAST	Calories	Totals
Orange juice (½ cup)	50	
Wheat Chex (¾ cup) + ½ cup skim milk + ½ banana	250	
Coffee	10	310 Cal
SNACK		
Fresh fruit in season (peach, plum, etc)	70	
Coffee or tea	10	80 Cal
LUNCH		
Soup (Appendix B - page 116)	100	
Small whole-grain roll	80	
Lettuce and sliced tomato with 1 Tbsp low-cal	45	
Unsweetened apple sauce (½ cup)	45	
Hot or iced tea	10	280 Cal
SNACK		
Popcorn Mini Bag	110	
Coffee or tea	10	120 Cal
DINNER		
Baked red snapper (Day 16 Recipe - page 95)	215	
Wild rice mix	160	
Green beans & tomato	75	
Yogurt (6 oz, nonfat, any flavor)	90	
Water	0	540 Cal
SNACK		
Two small cookies	160	
Coffee or tea	10	170 Cal
		1500 Cal

Day 17 – 1500 Calorie Meal Plan

BREAKFAST	Calories	Totals
Cantaloupe (½ medium)	50	
2 Fried eggs	160	
Toasted raisin bread (2 slices)	150	
Coffee	10	370 Cal
SNACK		
Yogurt (6 oz, nonfat, any flavor)	90	
Coffee or tea	10	100 Cal
LUNCH		
Soup (Appendix B - page 116)	160	
Lettuce & tomato sandwich (Tbsp light mayo)	170	
Gelatin dessert (unsweetened)	10	
Cucumber slices and carrots and celery sticks	15	
Hot or iced tea	10	365 Cal
SNACK		
Handful unsalted mixed nuts	100	
Coffee or tea	10	110 Cal
DINNER		
Tofu-Veggie Stir Fry (Day 17 Recipe - page 96)	230	
Whole-grain bread (1 slice)	70	
Fresh fruit in season (apple, peach, etc)	70	
Water with lemon section	10	380 Cal
SNACK		
Graham crackers (4 squares)	120	
Skim milk (4 oz)	45	165 Cal
		1490 Cal

Day 18 – 1500 Calorie Meal Plan

BREAKFAST	Calories	Totals
Grapefruit (½)	75	
Cheerios (1 cup) + ½ cup skim milk + about 15 raisins	190	
Coffee	10	275 Cal
SNACK		
Fresh fruit in season (peach, plum, etc)	70	
Coffee or tea	10	80 Cal
LUNCH		
Cottage cheese (1 cup low fat)	180	
Large green salad with 1½ Tbsp low-cal dressing	70	
Small whole-grain roll	80	
Hot or iced tea	10	340 Cal
SNACK		
Handful unsalted mixed nuts	100	
Coffee or tea	10	110 Cal
DINNER		
Grilled swordfish (Day 18 Recipe - page 97)	250	
Grilled potatoes	100	
Grilled cherry tomatoes	45	
Spinach (½ cup) steamed with garlic & drizzled	50	
Whole-grain bread (1 slice)	65	
Water with lemon section	15	525 Cal
SNACK		
Two small cookies	160	
Coffee or tea	10	170 Cal
		1500 Cal

Day 19 – 1500 Calorie Meal Plan

BREAKFAST	Calories	Totals
Cantaloupe (½ medium)	50	
Oatmeal (½ cup dry) + ½ cup skim milk + about 15 raisins	220	
Coffee	10	280 Cal
SNACK		
Fresh fruit in season (apple, plum, etc)	70	
Coffee or tea	10	80 Cal
LUNCH		
Grilled cheese sandwich (2 slices 2% cheese)	240	
Lettuce and sliced tomato	20	
Pickle spear	0	
Hot or iced tea	10	270 Cal
SNACK		
Popcorn Mini Bag	110	
Coffee or tea	10	120 Cal
DINNER		
Eat Out – vegetarian (Day 19 Recipe - page 98)		
Max allowable calories	630	630 Cal
SNACK		
100-Calorie Pack Cookies	100	
Coffee or tea	10	110 Cal
		1490 Cal

Day 20 – 1500 Calorie Meal Plan

BREAKFAST	Calories	Totals
Cantaloupe (½ medium)	50	
Shredded Wheat (1 cup) + ½ cup skim milk + ½ banana	260	
Coffee	10	320 Cal
SNACK		
Handful unsalted mixed nuts	100	
Coffee or tea	10	110 Cal
LUNCH		
Egg salad (1 egg + 1 Tbsp light mayo)	125	
Small whole-grain roll	80	
Lettuce & sliced tomato with 1 Tbsp low-cal	45	
Hot or iced tea	10	260 Cal
SNACK		
Yogurt (6 oz, nonfat, any flavor)	90	
Coffee or tea	10	100 Cal
DINNER		
Spaghetti alla Puttanesca (Day 20 Recipe - page 99)	345	
Large green salad with 1½ Tbsp low-cal dressing	70	
Italian or French bread (1 slice)	80	
Glass of red wine (4 oz)	100	
Water with lemon wedge	10	605 Cal
SNACK		
Graham crackers (4 squares)	120	
Coffee or tea	10	130 Cal
		1495 Cal

Day 21 – 1500 Calorie Meal Plan

BREAKFAST	Calories	Totals
Cantaloupe (½ medium)	50	
Oatmeal (½ cup dry) + ½ cup skim milk + about 15 raisins	220	
Whole-grain toast (1 slice)	70	
Coffee	10	350 Cal
SNACK		
Handful unsalted mixed nuts	100	
Coffee or tea	10	110 Cal
LUNCH		
Tuna salad (3 oz canned tuna, 1 tsp Evoo, onions, celery)	175	
Lettuce, tomato & Tbsp light mayo	35	
Small whole-grain roll	80	
Fresh fruit in season (peach, plum, etc)	70	
Water	0	360 Cal
SNACK		
Yogurt (6 oz, nonfat, any flavor)	90	90 Cal
DINNER		
Frozen Pasta-based dinner (Day 21 Recipe- page 100)	300	
Large green salad with 1½ Tbsp low-cal dressing	70	
Whole-grain bread (1 slice)	70	
Water	0	440 Cal
SNACK		
Dark chocolate (1 oz)	150	
Coffee or tea	10	160 Cal
		1510 Cal

Day 22 – 1500 Calorie Meal Plan

BREAKFAST	Calories	Totals
Fresh or frozen strawberries (½ cup)	25	
French toasted English Muffin (Day 2 Recipe - page 78)	270	
Light syrup (1 Tbsp)	30	
Coffee	10	335 Cal
SNACK		
Yogurt (6 oz, nonfat, any flavor)	90	
Coffee or tea	10	100 Cal
LUNCH		
Soup (Appendix B - page 116)	100	
Egg salad (1 egg + 1 Tbsp light mayo)	125	
Small whole-grain roll	80	
Hot or iced tea	10	315 Cal
SNACK		
Popcorn Mini Bag	110	
Coffee or tea	10	120 Cal
DINNER		
Tomato Risotto Salad (Day 22 Recipe - page 101)	310	
Whole-grain bread (1 slice)	70	
Fresh fruit in season (apple, peach, etc)	70	
Water with lemon wedge	10	520 Cal
SNACK		
100-Calorie Pack Cookies	100	
Coffee or tea	10	110 Cal
		1500 Cal

Day 23 – 1500 Calorie Meal Plan

BREAKFAST	Calories	Totals
Cantaloupe (½ medium)	50	
Shredded Wheat (1 cup) + ½ cup skim milk + ½ banana	260	
Coffee	10	320 Cal
SNACK		
Fresh fruit in season (apple, plum, etc)	70	
Coffee or tea	10	80 Cal
LUNCH		
Peanut butter (2 Tbsp) - 2 slices of whole-grain bread	340	
Hot or iced tea	10	350 Cal
SNACK		
Popcorn Mini Bag	110	
Coffee or tea	10	120 Cal
DINNER		
Beans & greens salad (Day 23 Recipe - page 102)	260	
Whole-grain bread (1 slice)	70	
Baked potato (medium)	100	
Fresh fruit in season (peach, plum, etc)	70	
Water with lemon section	10	510 Cal
SNACK		
100-Calorie Pack Cookies	100	
Coffee or tea	10	110 Cal
		1490 Cal

Day 24 – 1500 Calorie Meal Plan

BREAKFAST	Calories	Totals
Fresh orange sliced	75	
Soft-boiled egg	80	
Whole-grain toast (2 slices)	140	
Coffee	10	305 Cal
SNACK		
Yogurt (6 oz nonfat, any flavor)	90	
Coffee or tea	10	100 Cal
LUNCH		
Salad – 3 oz salmon, 1 tsp Evoo, onions & celery	200	
Lettuce & tomato wedges	20	
Rye bread (1 slice)	70	
Coffee or tea	10	300 Cal
SNACK		
Popcorn Mini Bag	110	
Coffee or tea	10	120 Cal
DINNER		
Four bean plus salad (1 cup) (Day 24 Recipe -page103)	270	
Baked potato (medium)	100	
Whole-grain bread (1 slice)	70	
Fresh fruit in season (apple, plum, etc)	70	
Water with lemon wedge	10	520 Cal
SNACK		
Kashi TLC Chewy Granola Bar	140	
Coffee or tea	10	150 Cal
		1505 Cal

Day 25 – 1500 Calorie Meal Plan

BREAKFAST	Calories	Totals
Grapefruit (½)	75	
Cheerios (1 cup) + ½ cup skim milk + about 15 raisins	190	
Whole grain toast (1 slice)	70	
Coffee	10	345 Cal
SNACK		
Fresh fruit in season (apple, peach, etc)	70	
Coffee or tea	10	80 Cal
LUNCH		
Cottage cheese (1 cup low fat)	180	
Large green salad with 1½ Tbsp low-cal dressing	70	
Small whole-grain roll	80	
Hot or iced tea	10	340 Cal
SNACK		
Yogurt (6 oz nonfat, any flavor)	90	90 Cal
DINNER		
Tofu with veggies & peanuts (Day 25 Recipe - page 104)	320	
Baked potato (medium)	100	
Small whole-grain roll	80	
Water	0	500 Cal
SNACK		
Kashi TLC Chewy Granola Bar	140	
Coffee or tea	10	150 Cal
		1505 Cal

Day 26 – 1500 Calorie Meal Plan

BREAKFAST	Calories	Totals
Cantaloupe (½ medium)	50	
Fried egg	80	
Whole-grain toast (2 slices)	140	
Coffee	10	280 Cal
SNACK		
Handful unsalted mixed nuts	100	
Coffee or tea	10	110 Cal
LUNCH		
Soup (Appendix B - page 116)*	280	
Hard whole-grain roll (medium)	80	
Lettuce & tomato slices	20	
Gelatin dessert (unsweetened)	10	
Hot or iced tea	10	400 Cal
* Enjoy 2 servings of 140 Cal soup.		
SNACK		
Fresh fruit in season (apple, plum, etc)	70	
Coffee or tea	10	80 Cal
DINNER		
Grilled scallops (Day 26 Recipe - page 105)	210	
Grilled polenta (Day 26 Recipe)	125	
Mushroom-steamed green beans-red onion,	55	
Yogurt (6 oz, nonfat, any flavor)	90	
Water with lemon section	10	490 Cal
SNACK		
Graham crackers (4 squares)	120	
Coffee or tea	10	130 Cal
		1490 Cal

Day 27 – 1500 Calorie Meal Plan

BREAKFAST	Calories	Totals
Cantaloupe (½ medium)	50	
Oatmeal (½ cup dry) + ½ cup skim milk + about 15 raisins	220	
Coffee	10	280 Cal
SNACK		
Fresh fruit in season (apple, plum, etc)	70	
Coffee or tea	10	80 Cal
LUNCH		
Two servings (1 cup) left over bean salad from Day 24	270	
Small whole-grain roll	80	
Lettuce & tomato slices	20	
Hot or iced tea	10	380 Cal
SNACK		
Yogurt (6 oz, nonfat, any flavor)	90	
Coffee or tea	10	100 Cal
DINNER		
Fettuccine (Day 27 Recipe - page 106)	290	
Large green salad with 1½ Tbsp low-cal dressing	70	
Italian or French bread (1 slice)	80	
Glass of red wine (4 oz)	100	
Water	0	540 Cal
SNACK		
100-Calorie Pack Cookies	100	
Coffee or tea	10	110 Cal
		1510 Cal

Day 28 – 1500 Calorie Meal Plan

BREAKFAST	Calories	Totals
Tomato juice (½ cup)	20	
Shredded Wheat (1 cup) + ½ cup skim milk + ½ banana	260	
Coffee	10	290 Cal
SNACK		
Handful unsalted mixed nuts	100	100 Cal
LUNCH		
Grilled Swiss cheese sandwich (2 oz low-fat cheese)	320	
Cucumber + tomato slices & 1 tsp low-cal dressing	30	
Hot or iced tea	10	360 Cal
SNACK		
Yogurt (6 oz, nonfat, any flavor)	90	
Coffee or tea	10	100 Cal
DINNER		
Frozen vegetarian dinner (Day 28 Recipe - page 107)	300	
Large green salad with 1½ Tbsp low-cal dressing	70	
Whole-grain bread (1 slice)	70	
Fresh fruit in season (peach, plum, etc)	70	
Water	0	520 Cal
SNACK		
Graham crackers (4 squares)	120	
Coffee or tea	10	130 Cal
		1500 Cal

Day 29 – 1500 Calorie Meal Plan

BREAKFAST	Calories	Totals
Orange juice (½ cup)	50	
Wild blueberry pancakes (Day 10 Recipe - page 86)	190	
Turkey bacon (2 slices)	70	
Light syrup (1½ Tbsp)	45	
Coffee	10	365 Cal
SNACK		
Handful unsalted mixed nuts	100	
Coffee or tea	10	110 Cal
LUNCH		
Salad (3 oz tuna, 1 tsp Evoo, onions & celery)	175	
Lettuce & tomato wedges, Rye bread (1 slice)	85	
Fresh fruit in season (pear, peach, etc)	70	
Coffee or tea	10	340 Cal
SNACK		
Fiber One Chocolate Fudge Brownie	90	
Coffee or tea	10	100 Cal
DINNER		
Barbequed shrimp (Day 29 Recipe - page 108)	160	
Corn on the cob (medium)	90	
Steamed broccoli (1 cup equivalent)	50	
Gelatin dessert (unsweetened)	10	
Yogurt (6 oz, nonfat, any flavor)	90	
Water with lemon section	10	410 Cal
SNACK		
Two small cookies	160	
Coffee or tea	10	170 Cal
		1505 Cal

Day 30 – 1500 Calorie Meal Plan

BREAKFAST	Calories	Totals
Fresh orange sliced	75	
Cheerios (1 cup) + ½ cup skim milk + about 15 raisins	190	
Whole grain toast (1 slice)	70	
Coffee	10	345 Cal
SNACK		
Fresh fruit in season (peach, plum, etc)	70	
Coffee or tea	10	80 Cal
LUNCH		
Soup (Appendix B - page 116)	220	
Large green salad with 1½ Tbsp low-cal dressing	70	
Small whole-grain roll	80	
Water	0	370 Cal
SNACK		
Handful unsalted mixed nuts	100	
Coffee or tea	10	110 Cal
DINNER		
Tofu steak with veggies (Day 30 Recipe - page 109)	275	
Small whole-grain roll	80	
Yogurt (6 oz nonfat, any flavor)	90	
Water	0	445 Cal
SNACK		
Kashi TLC Chewy Granola Bar	140	
Coffee or tea	10	150 Cal
		1500 Cal

1200-Calorie Daily Menus

Day 1 – 1200 Calorie Meal Plan

BREAKFAST	Calories	Totals
<u>Orange juice (½ cup)</u>	50	
Wheaties (¾ cup) + ½ cup skim milk + ½ banana	190	
Coffee (See page 12)	10	250 Cal
<u>SNACK</u>		
Fresh fruit in season (apple, peach, etc)	70	
Coffee or tea	10	80 Cal
<u>LUNCH</u>		
Soup (Appendix B - page 116)	60	
Sliced hard-boiled egg on 1 slice rye bread	150	
Lettuce & tomato slices	20	
Coffee or tea	10	240 Cal
<u>SNACK</u>		
One small cookie*	80	
Skim milk (4 oz)	40	120 Cal
<u>DINNER</u>		
Baked Herb-Crusted Cod (Day 1 Recipe - page 77)	230	
Spinach (½ cup) steamed with garlic & drizzled	100	
Asparagus (7 spear cooked & drained)	20	
Whole grain Bread -1 slice (See page 8)	65	
Water	0	415 Cal
<u>SNACK</u>		
Fiber One Chocolate Fudge Brownie	90	
Coffee or tea	10	100 Cal
* Oatmeal, ginger snap, sugar, etc - check calories!		1205 Cal

Day 2 – 1200 Calorie Meal Plan

BREAKFAST	Calories	Totals
Fresh or frozen strawberries (½ cup)	25	
French toasted English Muffin (Day 2 Recipe - page 78)	270	
Light syrup (1 Tbsp)	30	
Coffee	10	335 Cal
SNACK		
Coffee or tea	10	10 Cal
LUNCH		
Tuna salad (3 oz tuna, 1 tsp Evoo, onions & celery)	175	
Lettuce & tomato wedges	20	
Fresh fruit in season (apple, peach, etc)	70	
Hot or iced tea	10	275 Cal
SNACK		
Yogurt (6 oz, nonfat, any flavor)*	90	
Coffee or tea	10	100 Cal
DINNER		
Polenta-stuffed peppers (Day 2b Recipe - page 79)	290	
Large green salad with 1½ Tbsp low-cal	70	
Water with lemon wedge	10	370 Cal
** See page 7.		
SNACK		
Graham crackers (3 squares)	90	
Coffee or tea	10	100 Cal
* Such as Dannon Lite & Fit. Buy 32 oz container; use 6 oz.		1190 Cal

Day 3 – 1200 Calorie Meal Plan

BREAKFAST	Calories	Totals
Grapefruit (½)	75	
Scrambled egg (page 12)	80	
Whole-grain toast (1 slice) (page 9)	65	
Coffee	10	230 Cal
SNACK		
Coffee or tea	10	10 Cal
LUNCH		
Peanut butter (1 Tbsp) on 1 slice whole-grain bread	170	
Skim milk (4 oz)	45	
Fresh fruit in season (apple, peach, etc)	70	285 Cal
SNACK		
Popcorn Mini Bag*	110	
Coffee or tea	10	120 Cal
DINNER		
Crumbly-Tofu Scramble (Day 3 Recipe - page 80)	240	
Sautéed red peppers with onions	70	
Green beans (steamed) & mashed cauliflower	45	
Large green salad with 1½ Tbsp low-cal dressing	70	
Water with lemon wedge	10	435 Cal
SNACK		
Graham crackers (4 squares)	120	
Coffee or tea	10	130 Cal
* Such as Orville Redenbacher's Smart Pop		1210 Cal

Day 4 – 1200 Calorie Meal Plan

BREAKFAST	Calories	Totals
Grapefruit (½)	75	
Cheerios (1 cup) + ½ cup skim milk + about 15 raisins*	190	
Coffee	10	275 Cal
SNACK		
Coffee or tea	10	10 Cal
LUNCH		
Cottage cheese (1 cup low fat)	180	
Large green salad with 1½ Tbsp low-cal dressing	70	
Hot or iced tea	10	260 Cal
SNACK		
Fresh fruit in season (peach, plum, etc)	70	
Coffee or tea	10	80 Cal
DINNER		
Easy Penne Pasta (Day 4 Recipe - page 81)	375	
Italian or French bread (1 slice)	80	
Glass red wine (4 oz)	100	
Water	0	555 Cal
SNACK		
Coffee or tea	10	10 Cal
* See page 12 re substituting blueberries for raisins.		1190 Cal

Day 5 – 1200 Calorie Meal Plan

BREAKFAST	Calories	Totals
Cantaloupe (½ medium)	50	
Fried egg	80	
Toasted raisin bread (1 slice)	75	
Coffee	10	215 Cal
SNACK		
Coffee or tea	10	10 Cal
LUNCH		
Soup (Appendix B - page 116)	140	
Small whole-grain roll	80	
Lettuce and sliced tomato with 1 Tbsp low-cal	45	
Canned pineapple (½ cup, no-sugar-added juice)	40	
Hot or iced tea	10	315 Cal
SNACK		
Yogurt (6 oz, nonfat, any flavor)	90	
Coffee or tea	10	100 Cal
DINNER		
Frozen fish dinner (Day 5 Recipe - page 82)	340	
Large green salad with 1½ Tbsp low-cal dressing	70	
Water	0	410 Cal
SNACK		
Graham crackers (3 squares)	90	
Skim milk (6 oz)	60	150 Cal
		1200 Cal

Day 6 – 1200 Calorie Meal Plan

BREAKFAST	Calories	Totals
Tomato juice (½ cup)	20	
Shredded Wheat (1 cup) + ½ cup skim milk + ½ banana	265	
Coffee	10	295 Cal
SNACK		
Coffee or tea	10	10 Cal
LUNCH		
Salad – 3 oz canned salmon, 1 tsp Evoo, onions & celery	200	
Small whole-grain roll	80	
Lettuce	0	
Hot or iced tea	10	290 Cal
SNACK		
Yogurt (6 oz, nonfat, any flavor)	90	
Coffee or tea	10	100 Cal
DINNER		
Pizza (Day 6 Recipe - page 83)	350	
Large green salad with 1½ Tbsp low-cal dressing	70	
Fresh fruit in season (pear, plum, etc)	70	
Water	0	490 Cal
SNACK		
Coffee or tea	10	10 Cal
		1195 Cal

Day 7 – 1200 Calorie Meal Plan

BREAKFAST	Calories	Totals
Cantaloupe (½ medium)	50	
Oatmeal (½ cup dry) + ½ cup skim milk + about 15 raisins	220	
Coffee	10	280 Cal
SNACK		
Coffee or tea	10	10 Cal
LUNCH		
Grilled cheese sandwich (2 slices 2% cheese)	230	
Lettuce and sliced tomato	20	
Pickle spear	0	
Water	0	250 Cal
SNACK		
Carrot sticks + ¼ cup low-fat cottage cheese & chives	60	
Coffee or tea	10	70 Cal
DINNER		
Eat Out – Vegetarian (Day 7 Recipe - page 84)		
Max allowable calories	530	530 Cal
SNACK		
Graham crackers (2 squares)	60	
Coffee or tea	10	70 Cal
		1210 Cal

Day 8 – 1200 Calorie Meal Plan

BREAKFAST	Calories	Totals
Cantaloupe (½ medium)	50	
Wheaties (¾ cup) + ½ cup skim milk + ½ banana	190	
Coffee	10	250 Cal
SNACK		
Coffee or tea	10	10 Cal
LUNCH		
Soup (Appendix B - page 116)	130	
Lettuce & tomato sandwich + 1 Tbsp light mayo	150	
Hot or iced tea	10	290 Cal
SNACK		
Coffee or tea	10	10 Cal
DINNER		
Baked salmon with salsa (Day 8 Recipe - page 85)	215	
Summer squash, zucchini and tomatoes	60	
Brown rice (½ cup)	100	
Large green salad with 1½ Tbsp low-cal dressing	70	
Fresh fruit in season (apple, plum, etc)	70	
Water with lemon wedge	15	530 Cal
SNACK		
Popcorn Mini Bag	110	
Coffee or tea	10	120 Cal
		1210 Cal

Day 9 – 1200 Calorie Meal Plan

BREAKFAST	Calories	Totals
Orange juice (½ cup)	50	
Soft-boiled egg	80	
Whole-grain toast (1 slice)	65	
Coffee	10	205 Cal
SNACK		
Coffee or tea	10	10 Cal
LUNCH		
Tuna salad (3 oz tuna, 1 tsp Evoo, onions & celery)	175	
Lettuce & tomato wedges	20	
Rye bread (1 slice)	65	
Fresh fruit in season (pear, peach, etc)	70	
Coffee or tea	10	340 Cal
SNACK		
Yogurt (6 oz, nonfat, any flavor)	90	
Coffee or tea	10	100 Cal
DINNER		
Portobello mushroom burger (Day 9 Recipe -page 86)	270	
Lettuce and sliced tomato	20	
Whole-grain hard roll	140	
Steamed green beans	25	
Pickle spear	0	
Water with lemon wedge	10	465 Cal
SNACK		
One small cookie	80	
Coffee or tea	10	90 Cal
		1210 Cal

Day 10 – 1200 Calorie Meal Plan

BREAKFAST	Calories	Totals
Orange juice (½ cup)	50	
Wild blueberry pancakes (Day 10 Recipe - page 87)	190	
Light syrup (1½ Tbsp)	45	
Coffee	10	365 Cal
SNACK		
Coffee or tea	10	10 Cal
LUNCH		
Peanut butter (2 Tbsp) 2 slices of whole-grain bread	330	
Skim milk (4 oz)	45	375 Cal
SNACK		
Coffee or tea	10	10 Cal
DINNER		
Eggplant Parmesan (Day 10b Recipe - page 88)	270	
Large tossed salad with 1½ Tbsp low-cal dressing	70	
Italian or French bread (1 slice)	80	
Water	0	430 Cal
SNACK		
Coffee or tea	10	10 Cal
		1200 Cal

Day 11 – 1200 Calorie Meal Plan

BREAKFAST	Calories	Totals
Fresh sliced orange	75	
Cheerios (1 cup) + ½ cup skim milk + about 15 raisins	240	
Coffee	10	325 Cal
SNACK		
Handful unsalted mixed nuts	100	
Coffee or tea	10	110 Cal
LUNCH		
Cottage cheese (1 cup low fat)	180	
Large green salad with 1½ Tbsp low-cal dressing	70	
Small whole-grain roll	80	
Water	0	330 Cal
SNACK		
Coffee or tea	10	10 Cal
DINNER		
Mexican Beans and Rice (Day 11 Recipe - page 89)	270	
Whole-grain bread (1 slice)	70	
Fresh fruit in season (peach, plum, etc)	70	
Water with lemon wedge	10	420 Cal
SNACK		
Coffee or tea	10	10 Cal
		1205 Cal

Day 12 – 1200 Calorie Meal Plan

BREAKFAST	Calories	Totals
Grapefruit (½)	75	
Scrambled egg	80	
Whole-grain toast (1 slice)	65	
Coffee	10	230 Cal
SNACK		
Coffee or tea	10	10 Cal
LUNCH		
Soup (Appendix B - page 116)	140	
Tomato slices, ¼ cup chopped fresh basil + ½ tsp Evoo	40	
Whole-grain bread (1 slice)	65	
Hot or iced tea	10	255 Cal
SNACK		
Yogurt (6 oz, nonfat, any flavor)	90	
Coffee or tea	10	100 Cal
DINNER		
Eat Out – Fish dinner (Day 12 Recipe - page 90)		
Max allowable calories	595	595 Cal
SNACK		
Coffee or tea	10	10 Cal
		1200 Cal

Day 13 – 1200 Calorie Meal Plan

BREAKFAST	Calories	Totals
Orange juice (½ cup)	50	
Shredded Wheat (1 cup) + ½ cup skim milk + ½ banana	260	
Coffee	10	320 Cal
SNACK		
Coffee or tea	10	10 Cal
LUNCH		
Egg salad (1 egg + 1 Tbsp light mayo)	125	
Small whole-grain roll	80	
Hot or iced tea	10	315 Cal
SNACK		
Coffee or tea	10	10 Cal
DINNER		
Pasta w Marinara sauce (Day 13 Recipe - page 91)	225	
Large green salad with 1½ Tbsp low-cal dressing	70	
Fresh fruit in season (pear, plum, etc)	70	
Italian or French bread (1 slice)	80	
Water with lemon section	15	460 Cal
SNACK		
Fiber One Chocolate Fudge Brownie	90	
Coffee or tea	10	100 Cal
		1215 Cal

Day 14 – 1200 Calorie Meal Plan

BREAKFAST	Calories	Totals
Cantaloupe (½ medium)	50	
Low-Cal Smoothie (Day 14a Recipe - page 92)	220	
Coffee	10	280 Cal
SNACK		
Coffee or tea	10	10 Cal
LUNCH		
Grilled Swiss cheese sandwich (2 oz low-fat cheese)	310	
Pickle spear	0	
Hot or iced tea	10	320 Cal
SNACK		
Fresh fruit in season (apple, plum, etc)	70	70 Cal
DINNER		
Frozen Fish dinner (Day 14b Recipe - page 93)	300	
Large green salad with 1½ Tbsp low-cal dressing	70	
Water with lemon wedge	10	380 Cal
SNACK		
Graham crackers (4 squares)	120	
Coffee or tea	10	130 Cal
		1190 Cal

Day 15 – 1200 Calorie Meal Plan

BREAKFAST	Calories	Totals
Fresh or frozen strawberries (1 cup)	50	
French toast (made with 2 slices whole-grain	250	
Light syrup (1 Tbsp)	30	
Coffee	10	340 Cal
SNACK		
Coffee or tea	10	10 Cal
LUNCH		
Tuna salad (3 oz tuna, 1 tsp Evoo, onions & celery)	175	
Lettuce & tomato wedges	20	
Rye bread (1 slice)	65	
Coffee or tea	10	270 Cal
SNACK		
Yogurt (6 oz, nonfat, any flavor)	90	
Coffee or tea	10	100 Cal
DINNER		
Veggies with Couscous (Day 15 Recipe - page 94)	320	
Small whole-grain roll	80	
Fresh fruit in season (pear, plum, etc)	70	
Water	0	480 Cal
SNACK		
Coffee or tea	10	10 Cal
		1210 Cal

Day 16 – 1200 Calorie Meal Plan

BREAKFAST	Calories	Totals
Orange juice (½ cup)	50	
Wheat Chex (¾ cup) + ½ cup skim milk + ½ banana	250	
Coffee	10	310 Cal
SNACK		
Coffee or tea	10	10 Cal
LUNCH		
Soup (Appendix B - page 116)	100	
Small whole-grain roll	80	
Lettuce and sliced tomato with 1 Tbsp low-cal	45	
Hot or iced tea	10	235 Cal
SNACK		
Fresh fruit in season (apple, peach, etc)	70	
Coffee or tea	10	80 Cal
DINNER		
Baked red snapper (Day 16 Recipe - page 95)	215	
Wild rice mix	160	
Green beans & tomato	75	
Water with lemon section	15	465 Cal
SNACK		
Yogurt (6 oz, nonfat, any flavor)	90	
Coffee or tea	10	100 Cal
		1200 Cal

Day 17 – 1200 Calorie Meal Plan

BREAKFAST	Calories	Totals
Cantaloupe (½ medium)	50	
Fried egg	80	
Toasted raisin bread (1 slice)	75	
Coffee	10	215 Cal
SNACK		
Yogurt (6 oz, nonfat, any flavor)	90	90 Cal
LUNCH		
Soup (Appendix B - page 116)	150	
Lettuce & tomato sandwich (1 Tbsp light mayo)	170	
Cucumber slices and carrot & celery sticks	15	
Hot or iced tea	10	345 Cal
SNACK		
Handful unsalted mixed nuts	100	100 Cal
DINNER		
Tofu-Veggie Stir Fry (Day 17 Recipe - page 96)	230	
Whole-grain bread (1 slice)	70	
Fresh fruit in season (apple, peach, etc)	70	
Water with lemon section	10	380 Cal
SNACK		
Graham crackers (2 squares)	60	
Coffee or tea	10	70 Cal
		1200Cal

Day 18 – 1200 Calorie Meal Plan

BREAKFAST	Calories	Totals
Grapefruit (½)	75	
Cheerios (1 cup) + ½ cup skim milk + about 15 raisins	190	
Coffee	10	275 Cal
SNACK		
Coffee or tea	10	10 Cal
LUNCH		
Cottage cheese (1 cup low fat)	180	
Large green salad with 1½ Tbsp low-cal dressing	70	
Small whole-grain roll	80	
Hot or iced tea	10	340 Cal
SNACK		
Handful unsalted mixed nuts	100	
Coffee or tea	10	110 Cal
DINNER		
Grilled swordfish (Day 18 Recipe - page 97)	250	
Grilled potatoes	100	
Grilled cherry tomatoes	45	
Spinach (½ cup) steamed with garlic & drizzled	50	
Water with lemon section	10	455 Cal
SNACK		
Coffee or tea	10	10 Cal
		1200 Cal

Day 19 – 1200 Calorie Meal Plan

BREAKFAST	Calories	Totals
Grapefruit (½)	75	
Scrambled egg	80	
Whole-grain toast (1 slice)	65	
Coffee	10	230 Cal
SNACK		
Yogurt (6 oz nonfat, any flavor)	90	90 Cal
LUNCH		
Soup (Appendix B - page 116)*	100	
Grilled cheese ½ sandwich (1 slice 2% cheese)	120	
Water	0	220 Cal
SNACK		
Coffee or tea	10	10 Cal
DINNER		
Eat Out – Vegetarian (Day 19 Recipe - page 98)		
Max allowable calories	640	640 Cal
SNACK		
Coffee or tea	10	10 Cal
		1210 Cal

Day 20 – 1200 Calorie Meal Plan

BREAKFAST	Calories	Totals
Tomato juice (½ cup)	20	
Shredded Wheat (1 cup) + ½ cup skim milk + ½ banana	260	
Coffee	10	290 Cal
SNACK		
Handful unsalted mixed nuts	100	
Coffee or tea	10	110 Cal
LUNCH		
Egg salad (1 egg + 1 Tbsp light mayo)	125	
Small whole-grain roll	80	
Lettuce & sliced tomato with 1 Tbsp low-cal	45	
Hot or iced tea	10	260 Cal
SNACK		
Yogurt (6 oz, nonfat, any flavor)	90	
Coffee or tea	10	100 Cal
DINNER		
Spaghetti alla Puttanesca (Day 20 Recipe - page 99)	345	
Large green salad with 1½ Tbsp low-cal dressing	70	
Water with lemon section	15	430 Cal
SNACK		
Coffee or tea	10	10 Cal
		1200 Cal

Day 21 – 1200 Calorie Meal Plan

BREAKFAST	Calories	Totals
Cantaloupe (½ medium)	50	
Oatmeal (½ cup dry) + ½ cup skim milk + about 15 raisins	220	
Coffee	10	280 Cal
SNACK		
Coffee or tea	10	10 Cal
LUNCH		
Tuna salad (3 oz canned tuna, 1 tsp Evoo, onions, celery)	175	
Lettuce, tomato & Tbsp light mayo	35	
Small whole-grain roll	80	
Fresh fruit in season (peach, plum, etc)	70	
Water	0	360 Cal
SNACK		
Yogurt (6 oz, nonfat, any flavor)	90	
Coffee or tea	10	100 Cal
DINNER		
Frozen Pasta meal (Day 21 Recipe - page 100)	300	
Large green salad with 1½ Tbsp low-cal dressing	70	
Whole-grain bread (1 slice)	70	
Water with lemon section	10	450 Cal
SNACK		
Coffee or tea	10	10 Cal
		1210 Cal

Day 22 – 1200 Calorie Meal Plan

BREAKFAST	Calories	Totals
Fresh or frozen strawberries (1 cup)	25	
French toasted English Muffin (Day 2 Recipe - page 78)	270	
Light syrup (1 Tbsp)	30	
Coffee	10	335 Cal
SNACK		
Coffee or tea	10	10 Cal
LUNCH		
Soup (Appendix B - page 116)	160	
Egg salad (1 egg + 1 Tbsp light mayo)	125	
Small whole-grain roll	80	
Hot or iced tea	10	375 Cal
SNACK		
Coffee or tea	10	10 Cal
DINNER		
Tomato Risotto Salad (Day 22 Recipe - page 101)	310	
Whole-grain bread (1 slice)	65	
Large green salad with 1½ Tbsp low-cal dressing	70	
Water with lemon wedge	10	455 Cal
SNACK		
Coffee or tea	10	10 Cal
		1195 Cal

Day 23 – 1200 Calorie Meal Plan

BREAKFAST	Calories	Totals
Cantaloupe (½ medium)	50	
Wheaties (¾ cup) + ½ cup skim milk + ½ banana	190	
Coffee	10	250 Cal
SNACK		
Coffee or tea	10	10 Cal
LUNCH		
Peanut butter (2 Tbsp) 2 slices of whole-grain bread	340	
Hot or iced tea	10	350 Cal
SNACK		
Popcorn Mini Bag	110	
Coffee or tea	10	120 Cal
DINNER		
Beans & greens salad (Day 23 Recipe - page 102)	260	
Baked potato (medium)	100	
Fresh fruit in season (apple, peach, etc)	70	
Water with lemon wedge	10	440 Cal
SNACK		
Coffee or tea	10	10 Cal
		1180 Cal

Day 24 – 1200 Calorie Meal Plan

BREAKFAST	Calories	Totals
Fresh orange sliced	75	
Soft-boiled egg	80	
Whole-grain toast (1 slice)	70	
Coffee	10	235 Cal
SNACK		
Yogurt (6 oz, nonfat, any flavor)	90	
Coffee or tea	10	100 Cal
LUNCH		
Salad – 3 oz salmon, 1 tsp Evoo, onions & celery	200	
Lettuce & tomato wedges	20	
Rye bread (1 slice)	70	
Coffee or tea	10	300 Cal
SNACK		
Fresh fruit in season (pear, plum, etc)	70	
Coffee or tea	10	80 Cal
DINNER		
Four bean salad (1 cup) (Day 24 Recipe - page 103)	270	
Baked potato (medium)	100	
Whole-grain bread (1 slice)	70	
Water	10	450 Cal
SNACK		
Graham cracker (1 square)	30	
Coffee or tea	10	40 Cal
		1205 Cal

Day 25 – 1200 Calorie Meal Plan

BREAKFAST	Calories	Totals
Grapefruit (½)	75	
Cheerios (1 cup) + ½ cup skim milk + about 15 raisins	190	
Coffee	10	275 Cal
SNACK		
Coffee or tea	10	10 Cal
LUNCH		
Cottage cheese (1 cup low fat)	180	
Large green salad with 1½ Tbsp low-cal dressing	70	
Small whole-grain roll	80	
Hot or iced tea	10	340 Cal
SNACK		
Fresh fruit in season (peach, plum, etc)	70	70 Cal
DINNER		
Tofu w veggies & peanuts (Day 25 Recipe page 104)	320	
Baked potato (medium)	100	
Small whole-grain roll	80	
Water	0	500 Cal
SNACK		
Coffee or tea	10	10 Cal
		1205 Cal

Day 26 – 1200 Calorie Meal Plan

BREAKFAST	Calories	Totals
Cantaloupe (½ medium)	50	
Fried eggs (2 eggs)	160	
Toasted whole-grain bread (1 slice)	70	
Coffee	10	290 Cal
SNACK		
Yogurt (6 oz, nonfat, any flavor)	90	
Coffee or tea	10	100 Cal
LUNCH		
Soup (Appendix B - page 116)*	150	
Hard whole-grain roll (medium)	80	
Lettuce & tomato slices	20	
Hot or iced tea	10	260 Cal
SNACK		
Fresh fruit in season (apple, plum, etc)	70	
Coffee or tea	10	80 Cal
DINNER		
Grilled scallops (Day 26 Recipe - page 105)	210	
Grilled polenta (Day 26 Recipe)	125	
Mushroom-steamed green beans-red onion	45	
Grilled asparagus	10	
Large tossed salad with 1½ Tbsp low-cal dressing	70	
Water	0	460 Cal
SNACK		
Coffee or tea	10	10 Cal
		1200 Cal

Day 27 – 1200 Calorie Meal Plan

BREAKFAST	Calories	Totals
Cantaloupe (½ medium)	50	
Oatmeal (½ cup dry) + ½ cup skim milk + about 15 raisins	220	
Coffee	10	280 Cal
SNACK		
Fresh fruit in season (pear, plum, etc)	70	
Coffee or tea	10	80 Cal
LUNCH		
Two servings (1 cup) left over bean salad from Day 24	270	
Small whole-grain roll	80	
Lettuce & tomato slices	20	
Hot or iced tea	10	380 Cal
SNACK		
Coffee or tea	10	10 Cal
DINNER		
Fettuccine (Day 27 Recipe - page 106)	290	
Large green salad with 1½ Tbsp low-cal dressing	70	
Italian or French bread (1 slice)	80	
Water	0	440 Cal
SNACK		
Coffee or tea	10	10 Cal
		1200 Cal

Day 28 – 1200 Calorie Meal Plan

BREAKFAST	Calories	Totals
Cantaloupe (½ medium)	50	
Fried egg	80	
Toasted whole-grain bread (1 slice)	70	
Coffee	10	210 Cal
SNACK		
Yogurt (6 oz nonfat, any flavor)	90	90 Cal
LUNCH		
Soup (Appendix B - page 116)	140	
Small whole-grain roll	80	
Hot or iced tea	10	230 Cal
SNACK		
Popcorn Mini Bag	110	100 Cal
DINNER		
Frozen dinner (Day 28 Recipe - page 107)	300	
Large green salad with 1½ Tbsp low-cal dressing	70	
Whole-grain bread (1 slice)	70	
Fresh fruit in season (peach, plum, etc)	70	
Water	0	550 Cal
SNACK		
Coffee or tea	10	10 Cal
		1200 Cal

Day 29 – 1200 Calorie Meal Plan

BREAKFAST	Calories	Totals
Orange juice (½ cup)	50	
Wild blueberry pancakes (Day 10 Recipe - page 87)	190	
Turkey bacon (1 slice)	35	
Light syrup (1 Tbsp)	30	
Coffee	10	315 Cal
SNACK		
Yogurt (6 oz, nonfat, any flavor)	90	
Coffee or tea	10	100 Cal
LUNCH		
Salad (3 oz tuna, 1 tsp Evoo, onions & celery)	175	
Lettuce & tomato wedges	20	
Rye bread (1 slice)	65	
Fresh fruit in season (apple, peach, etc)	70	
Coffee or tea	10	340 Cal
SNACK		
Coffee or tea	10	10 Cal
DINNER		
Barbequed shrimp (Day 29 Recipe - page 108)	160	
Corn on the cob (medium)	90	
Steamed broccoli (1 cup equivalent)	50	
Water with lemon section	15	315 Cal
SNACK		
Popcorn Mini Bag	110	
Coffee or tea	10	120 Cal
		1200 Cal

Day 30 – 1200 Calorie Meal Plan

BREAKFAST	Calories	Totals
Fresh orange sliced	75	
Wheat Chex (¾ cup) + ½ cup skim milk + ½ banana	250	
Coffee	10	335 Cal
SNACK		
Coffee or tea	10	10 Cal
LUNCH		
Soup (Appendix B - page 116)	130	
Small whole-grain roll	80	
Raw zucchini slices, celery and carrot sticks	20	
Canned pineapple (½ cup, no-sugar-added juice)	40	
Hot or iced tea	10	280 Cal
SNACK		
Coffee or tea	10	10 Cal
DINNER		
Tofu steak with veggies (Day 30 Recipe - page 109)	275	
Small whole-grain roll	80	
Yogurt (6 oz nonfat, any flavor)	90	
Water	0	445 Cal
SNACK		
100-Calorie Pack Cookies*	100	
Coffee or tea	10	110 Cal
* Such as Nabisco Oreo/Chips Ahoy/etc		1190 Cal

Recipes & Diet Tips

Day 1 Recipe

Baked Herb-Crusted Cod

4 cod fish fillets (4 to 5 ounces each)
2 tablespoons flour
2 tablespoons cornmeal
2 tablespoons minced fresh herbs
2 teaspoons lemon juice

Sprinkle cod with lemon juice. Mix flour, cornmeal and herbs and dust the cod with the cornmeal-herb mixture. Bake in oven at 375 °F for 10 minutes. Add salt and black pepper to taste.
Serves 4. One serving is about 230 Calories (for cod only).

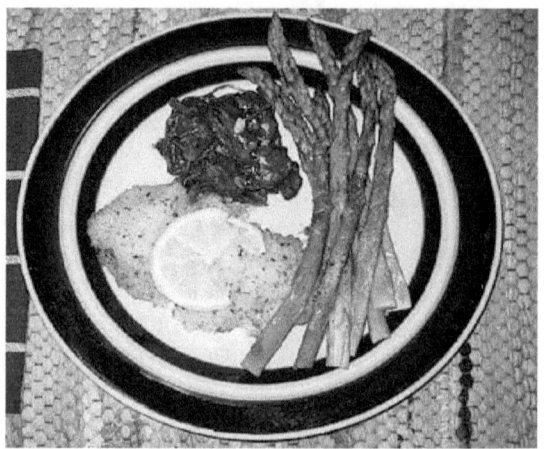

Diet Tip of the Day:. A **reducing diet is best supervised by a physician**. This is especially true when a great deal of weight needs to be lost, or if you have an ailment or a history of medical problems.

Day 2a Recipe
French-Toasted English Muffin
6 whole grain English muffins (light)
4 eggs
2 cups skim milk
2 teaspoons (tsp) vanilla
Dash of cinnamon

In a medium bowl, beat together eggs and skim milk. Add vanilla and cinnamon. Separate English muffins into halves and saturate slices in egg mixture. In a non-stick skillet coated with cooking spray, cook muffins until both sides are golden brown. Dust lightly with confectionary sugar. Serve hot or keep in an oven or warmer at 200 °F until ready to plate. **Serves 4**. Three English muffin slices (1½ muffins) per serving. Serving is 270 Calories.

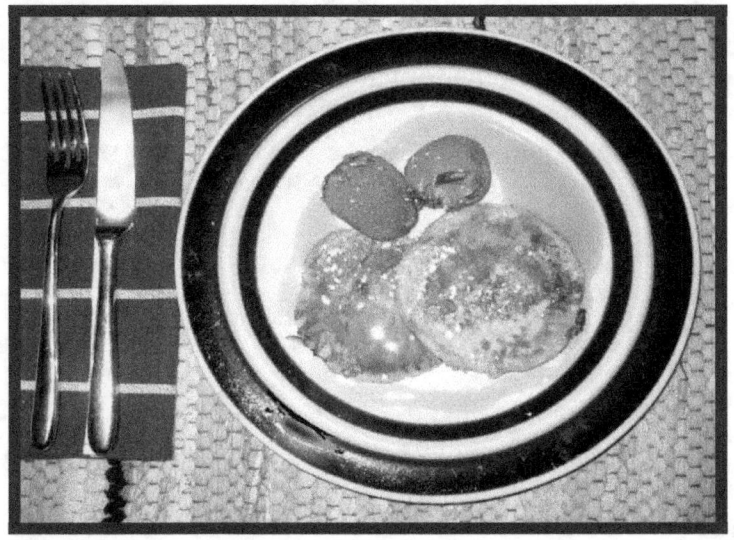

Diet Tip of the Day: **"Eat Slowly"** This is especially vital when you are trying to lose weight. If you are someone who eats fast, who finishes before everyone else at the table, you are not giving yourself a chance to feel full. While everyone else is still eating, you either sit there and pick, or you have seconds, taking in extra calories you could avoid if you would just slow down.

Day 2b Recipe

Polenta-Stuffed Peppers

4 plum tomatoes, halved
1 red onion, cut into wedges
1 tablespoon olive oil
4 poblano peppers, halved lengthwise and seeded
¼ teaspoon ground cinnamon
½ cup instant polenta
1 10-ounce package frozen corn
¼ cup soft goat cheese (2 ounces)
4 scallions, sliced
kosher salt and black pepper

1. Heat broiler. On a rimmed baking sheet, toss the tomatoes, onion, and oil. Turn tomatoes cut-side down. Add the peppers, cut-side down. Broil until tender and charred, stirring the onions and turning tomatoes and peppers halfway through, 5 to 8 minutes.
2. Heat oven to 400° F. In a food processor, puree tomatoes, onion, cinnamon, ½ teaspoon salt, and ¼ teaspoon pepper until smooth. Spread half the sauce in a 9-by-13-inch baking dish. Arrange the peppers in the dish, cut-side up.
3. In a medium saucepan, bring 2¼ cups water to a boil. Add ½ teaspoon salt. Gradually whisk in polenta. Cook, whisking constantly, until thickened, 3 to 4 minutes. Stir in corn, cheese, and all but 2 tablespoons of the scallions.
4. Divide the polenta among peppers. Top with remaining sauce and bake until heated through, 5 to 10 minutes. Sprinkle with the remaining scallions before serving.

Serves 4. 290 Calories per serving

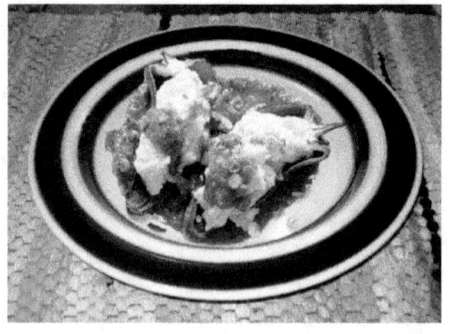

Day 3 Recipe

Crumbly-Tofu Scramble

16 ounces water-packed extra firm tofu
4 cups kale, chopped
3 tablespoons sesame oil
½ medium red onion, thinly sliced
1 medium red pepper, thinly sliced
1 teaspoon sea salt
1 teaspoon garlic powder
1 teaspoon cumin powder
½ teaspoon chili powder

For tofu draining and preparation tips go to page 113. While tofu is draining, prepare sauce by adding garlic, cumin and chili powder to a small bowl and adding enough water to make a pourable sauce. Set aside.

Warm a large skillet over medium heat. Add 2 tablespoons sesame oil, onion and red pepper. Season with a pinch of salt and pepper and stir. Cook until softened - about 5 minutes. Add kale, season with a bit more salt and pepper, and cover to steam for about 2 minutes.

Meanwhile, unwrap tofu and use a fork to crumble into bite-sized pieces. Use a spatula to move the veggies to one side of the pan and add tofu. Sauté for 2 minutes, then add sauce, pouring it mostly over the tofu and a little over the veggies. Stir immediately, evenly distributing the sauce. Cook for another 5 to 7 minutes.

<u>Serves 4</u>. About 250 Calories per serving (not including potatoes).

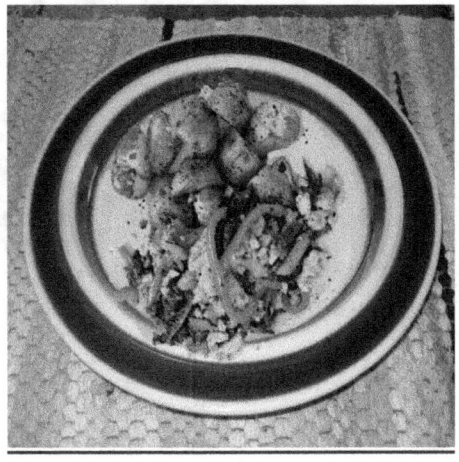

Day 4 Recipe

Easy Penne Pasta

1 16-ounce box whole-wheat penne pasta
1 tablespoon olive oil
¼ teaspoon red pepper flakes
1 24-ounce jar tomato-basil sauce
½ cup Parmesan cheese, grated
½ cup Italian parsley leaves, chopped

1. Bring a large pot of lightly salted water to a boil.
2. Meanwhile heat tomato-basil sauce and stir in red pepper flakes.
3. Cook the pasta according to package directions, drain and toss with tomato sauce. If desired, thin sauce with pasta water. Stir in olive oil before serving.
4. Sprinkle each serving with Parmesan cheese, parsley and salt to taste.

<u>Serves 6.</u> About 375 Calories per serving

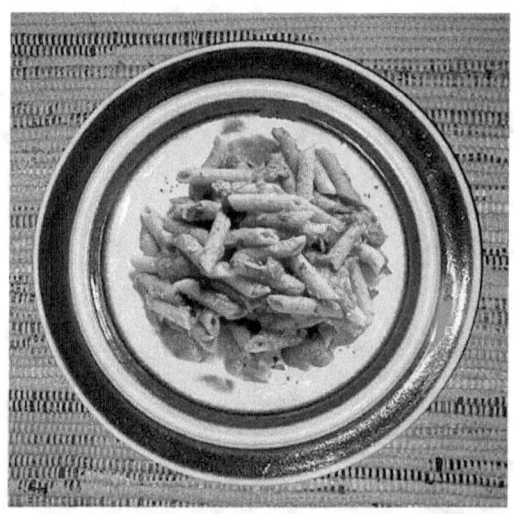

<u>Diet Tip of the Day:</u> **Take a daily multi-vitamin/mineral supplement.** This is very important when you're on a diet – as a kind of insurance policy.

Day 5 Recipe
Frozen-Fish Dinner
No recipe today. No cooking today. It's your day off! Some reasonably good frozen fish dinners are:
- Lean Cuisine Shrimp Alfredo (200 Cal)
- Lean Cuisine Szechuan Style Stir Fry with Shrimp (240 Cal)
- Lean Cuisine Salmon with Basil (250 Cal)
- Smart Ones Dragon Shrimp Lo Mien (240 Cal)

That's it. There are just not that many frozen fish dinners for sale at supermarkets. If you choose "Salmon with Lemon Dill Sauce" or "Shrimp with Vegetables," you will not use all of the **340 Calories allocated for this Day 5 meal**. In this case, use the excess 100 or so calories anyway you wish. Splurge on extra dessert or save the calories for the next day and have a larger piece of pizza!

Please read the important **Frozen-Food Safety Warning** in **Appendix C** page 117.

Diet Tip of the Day: **Buy a pedometer** and start walking. For the average person 2,100 steps amounts to walking about one mile. A Harvard study has shown that 8,000 to 10,000 step per day promote weight loss. And you're not obliged to walk continuously until you accrue all 10,000 steps. Rather, all steps throughout the day to wherever and whenever count toward your daily total. Because 10,000 steps a day may not be achievable by some people, particularly those who are elderly, sedentary, or who have chronic diseases, rather than insisting on a blanket 10,000 steps per day, your initial stepping goal should your baseline steps plus an increment of an additional 2,500 steps. (Your baseline being the number of steps you take in an average day.)

Day 6 Recipe

Grandma's Pizza

The following is a pizza recipe used by my Italian grandmother. She was from a small mountain village located between Rome and Naples.

Pizza dough: To save time use prepared dough, preferably whole grain. Flour a large cutting board. <u>Divide one pound of prepared pizza dough into four parts.</u> Roll out each dough ball as thin as possible.

Tomato sauce: Sauté ½ small onion, chopped fine, in 1 tsp olive oil. Add two finely chopped garlic cloves, 1½ cups chopped plum tomatoes and ½ tsp chopped fresh oregano. Stir and cook about 5 minutes on a low flame.

Pizza preparation & cooking: On each pizza, spread evenly about ¼ cup of the tomato sauce. Add about ½ ounce of shredded part-skim mozzarella cheese, 1 tsp Parmesan cheese, 3 slices of a Portobello mushroom, some torn fresh basil, and drizzle with Evoo. Put pizzas on a pan and place in 475 °F oven for about 15 to 20 minutes, or until crust is crisp and cheese is just melting. (Freeze left over sauce for use on Day 13.)

<u>Serves 4</u>. Make four pizzas. Each pizza contains about 350 Calories.

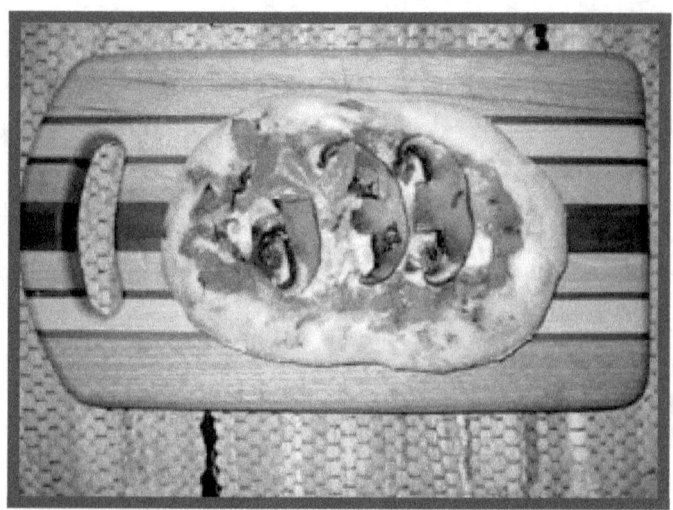

<u>Diet Tip of the Day:</u> For **life-long weight control** take a vigorous 30 to 60 minute walk everyday! That's right – everyday. Make exercise a nonflexible top priority part of your life. When it comes to exercise the key words are consistent, persistent, unyielding, dogged. Get the point?

Day 7 Recipe

Vegetarian Dinner - Out

No recipe today. No cooking today. Have dinner at your favorite vegetarian restaurant, but make sure you choose a restaurant where you have a fighting chance to achieve your calorie goal. For your vegetarian dinner out, your maximum allowable calories (including appetizer, soup, main course and dessert) are as follows:
- For the **1200 Calorie Diet**: 530 Calories
- For the **1500 Calorie Diet**: 630 Calories

Tips for Eating Vegetarian Out: First, order simple such as tofu stir fried with vegetables, and brown rice. Tell the waiter you want little to no added sauce or gravy. Estimate the calories in the meal: tofu is about 75 Calories per ounce, most vegetable servings average approximately 50 Calories per cup, rice is about 100 Calories per ½ cup, and add about 150 Calories for the oil used in the stir fry. Then knowing your allowable calorie total for the meal, decide how much to eat – and take the remainder home. If fresh fruit is not an option, pass on dessert and have the evening snack specified for that day on this diet.

In a restaurant, most nutritionists recommend you eat the low-calorie items on your plate first. Start with the salad, soup and veggies. By the time you get to the legumes and starches you will hopefully be full enough to be content with smaller portions of the higher-calorie choices.

Incidentally, if you live in a small town with no vegetarian restaurant, to stay on this diet, have a frozen vegetarian entree. And try to abide by the allowable calorie total.

Finally, some dieticians advise their dieting clients not to eat out. That's right. They believe eating at home is safer. But our thought is you have to eat out eventually so why not learn how while your resolve is high?

Diet Tip of the Day: When you're on a diet, eating in a restaurant can be a challenge, because most restaurant portions are huge, and can easily total more than 1,000 Calories. When eating in a restaurant decide how much to eat – and take the remainder home. A good general rule of thumb is to **eat half and bring the rest home**.

Day 8 Recipe
Baked Salmon with Salsa

This is a simple, straight-forward recipe. Again, the advantage of a simple recipe is there are no hidden calories.

    4 5 oz salmon fillets
    6 Tbsp bottled tomato-pepper salsa

Brown salmon fillets in non-stick pan and place in baking dish. Put fillets in an oven preheated to 350 °F for about 10 minutes. Plate the salmon. Stir prepared tomato-pepper salsa and spoon it over the salmon.

Serves 4. One salmon fillet is about 215 Calories.

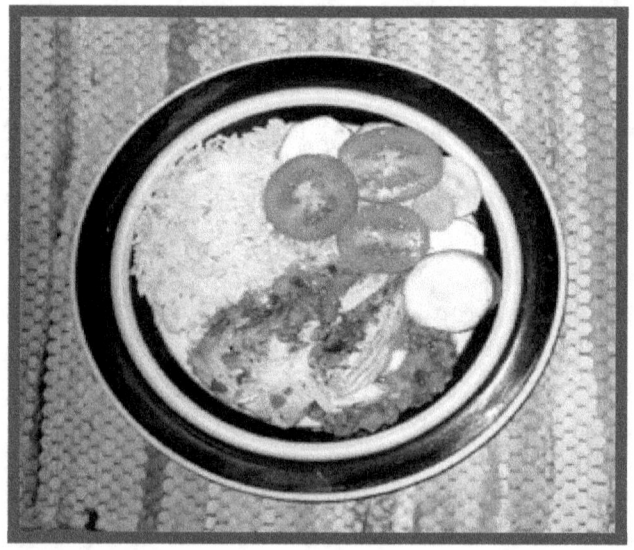

Diet Tip of the Day: **Have soup more often.** Most non-cream-based soups are filling and low-calorie.

Day 9 Recipe
Portobello Mushroom Burger

¼ cup low-sodium soy sauce
¼ cup balsamic vinegar
2 tablespoons olive oil
3 garlic cloves, minced
4 (4-inch) portobello mushroom caps
1 small red bell pepper
¼ cup light mayonnaise
½ teaspoon olive oil
⅛ teaspoon ground red pepper
4 (2-ounce) sandwich buns
4 (¼-inch-thick) slices tomato
4 curly leaf lettuce leaves

1. Combine first 4 ingredients in a large zip-top plastic bag; add mushrooms to bag. Seal and marinate at room temperature for 2 hours, turning bag occasionally. Remove mushrooms from bag. Start grill to medium heat.
3. Cut bell pepper in half lengthwise; discard seeds and membranes. Place pepper halves on grill rack coated with cooking spray; grill 15 minutes or until blackened, turning occasionally. Place in a zip-top plastic bag; seal. Let stand 10 minutes. Peel. Finely chop 1 pepper half; place in a small bowl. Add mayonnaise, ½ teaspoon oil, and ground red pepper; stir well.
4. Place mushrooms, gill sides down, on grill rack coated with cooking spray; grill 4 minutes on each side. Place buns, cut sides down, on grill rack coated with cooking spray; grill 30 seconds on each side or until toasted. Spread 2 tablespoons mayonnaise mixture on top half of each bun. Place 1 mushroom on bottom half of each bun. Top each mushroom with 1 tomato slice and 1 lettuce leaf.

Serves 4. About 270 Calories per serving.

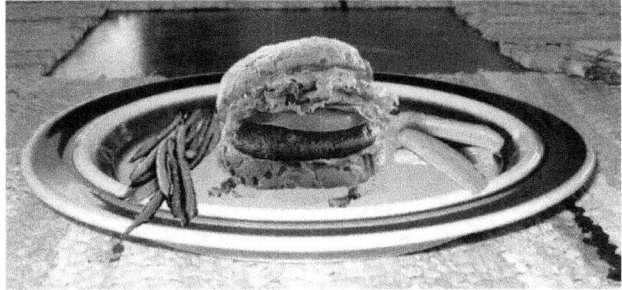

Day 10a Recipe
Wild Blueberry Pancakes
This recipe makes a relatively low calorie, wholesome batch of delicious
wild blueberry-whole grain-buttermilk pancakes.

    1 cup whole-grain flour
    1 cup buttermilk
    1 egg
    1 Tbsp vegetable oil
    1 tsp baking powder
    ½ tsp baking soda

Stir ingredients until blended. Add ¾ cup blueberries and gently stir.
Using medium heat, preheat a non-stick skillet coated with cooking spray.
Pour slightly less than ¼ cup of batter onto skillet per pancake. Cook
slowly until bubbles break on surface of pancake. Turn and cook until
other side is lightly browned. Makes 8 pancakes.

Pictured below are wild-blueberry pancakes with two slices of turkey
bacon.

Serves 4. Each pancake is about 95 Calories

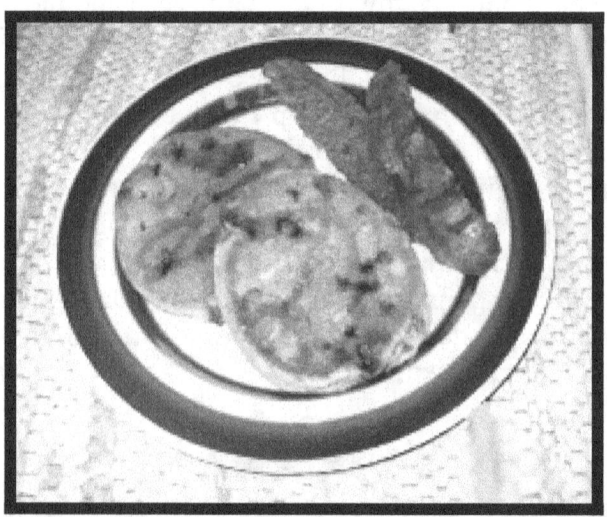

Diet Tip of the Day: A peanut butter sandwich on whole grain bread
with a glass of skim milk and an apple makes a nutritious, reasonably low-
calorie lunch.

Day 10b Recipe
Lo-Cal Eggplant Parmesan

3 medium eggplants, cut crosswise into ½-inch slices
3 tablespoons olive oil
1 large onion, finely chopped
1 large clove garlic, thinly sliced
1½ teaspoons dried oregano
1 28-ounce can no-salt plum tomatoes or crushed tomatoes
1 tablespoon red wine vinegar
½ cup (packed) fresh basil leaves
½ cup freshly grated Parmesan cheese
⅓ cup fine dry bread crumbs

1. Preheat oven to 450°F. Brush both sides of eggplant slices with olive oil, and place in a single layer on baking sheets. Bake until undersides are golden brown, 10 to 15 minutes, then turn and bake until other sides are lightly browned. Set aside. Reduce oven to 375°F.
2. Meanwhile, in a large saucepan over medium heat, add 2 tablespoons olive oil, onion, oregano and garlic. Sauté until soft, about 10 minutes. Add plum tomatoes and their juices. Break up whole tomatoes. Cover, reduce heat to low and simmer 15 to 20 minutes.
3. Add vinegar, basil and salt and pepper to taste. In a 10-by-6-inch baking pan, spoon a small amount of tomato sauce, then add a thin scattering of parmesan cheese, then a single layer of eggplant. Repeat until all ingredients are used, ending with a little sauce and a sprinkling of parmesan cheese. In a small bowl, combine bread crumbs with enough olive oil to moisten. Sprinkle on top.
4. Bake until eggplant mixture is bubbly and center is hot, 30 to 45 minutes depending on size of pan and thickness of layers. Remove from heat and allow to rest before serving.
<u>**Serves 5.**</u>   About 270 Calories per serving

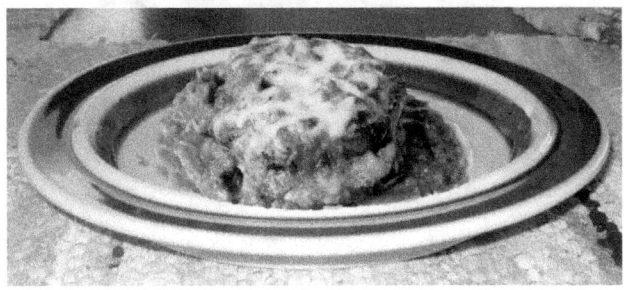

Day 11 Recipe

Mexican Rice and Beans

1 cup brown rice
½ small onion, diced
2 garlic cloves, minced
2 tablespoons olive oil
1 14½-ounce can diced tomatoes
1 15-ounce can black beans, rinsed and drained
1 medium fresh jalapeño, cored and finely chopped
½ cup finely chopped fresh oregano and cilantro leaves
½ teaspoon cumin, salt & pepper

1. In 1-quart saucepan, combine rice with 2 cups cold water. Bring to boil over medium-high heat, cover, reduce heat to low, and cook for 20 minutes. Remove from heat and let pan stand, covered, for another 5 minutes.

2. While rice steams, set a fine sieve over bowl and drain can of tomatoes. Pour tomato juices into a 1-cup liquid measure. Add enough water to tomato juices to equal 1 cup.

3. Heat a 10- to 12-inch skillet over medium-high heat. Pour in oil and stir-fry garlic and jalapeño until garlic browns and jalapeño smells pungent, about 1 minute. Add black beans, salt, and cumin; stir three times to incorporate mixture. Cook about 30 seconds.

4. Stir in tomato juice and water mixture and bring to a boil. Adjust heat to maintain a gentle boil and cook, stirring occasionally, until beans absorb much of liquid, about 6 minutes. Add tomatoes, oregano, cilantro, and cooked rice and cook, stirring occasionally, until rice is warm, about 2 minutes. Serve immediately.

Serves 6. About 270 Calories per serving

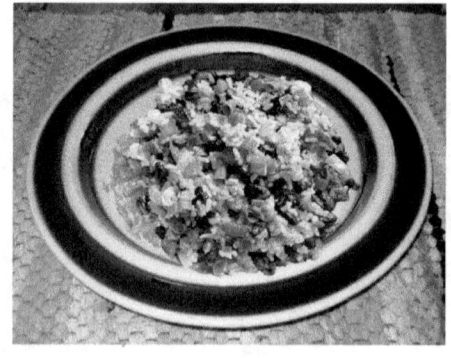

Day 12 Recipe

Fish Dinner - Out

No recipe today. No cooking today. Have a fish dinner at your favorite restaurant, but make sure you choose a restaurant where you have a good chance to achieve your calorie goal. For Day 12, your **goal for dinner is a maximum of 595 Calories**. This includes appetizer, soup, main course and dessert.

Tips for Eating Out: The following is almost an exact repeat of advice given for Day 7. First, order simple, such as broiled fish with steamed vegetables and brown rice. Tell the waiter you want no sauce, no gravy, nothing added. Then, knowing your calorie objective, and that fish is about 50 Calories per ounce, most steamed vegetable servings average approximately 50 Calories per cup, and rice is about 100 Calories per ½ cup, decide how much to eat – and take the remainder home. If fresh fruit is not an option, pass on dessert and have the evening snack specified for that day in the diet.

In a restaurant, I recommend you eat the low-calorie items on your plate first. Start with the salad, soup and veggies. By the time you get to the fish and starches you will hopefully be full enough to be content with smaller portions of the higher-calorie choices.

Diet Tip of the Day: Phytonutrients are found in plant foods such as fruits, vegetables, whole grains, dried beans, nuts and seeds. Unlike protein, fat, vitamins and minerals, phytonutrients are not necessary for life, but evidence is growing that phytonutrients have many beneficial qualities.

Day 13 Recipe

Pasta with Marinara Sauce

Prepare the sauce as you did for the Day 6 pizza. But because the pizza sauce is a bit too thick, add ¼ cup of pasta liquid to thin it. (The spiral pasta shape shown below is called Fusilli, and is a favorite because all the ridges really hold the sauce.)

> ½ pound <u>whole-grain</u> pasta
> ¼ tsp salt

Prepare the marinara tomato sauce as per Day 6 sauce but dilute it with ¼ cup of pasta liquid. Bring 2 quarts of lightly salted water to a boil. Add pasta and stir occasionally (to keep pasta from sticking to the bottom of the pot). Keep water boiling and cook until pasta are "al dente." (Cooking time is approximately 9 minutes.) Drain pasta, add marinara sauce and serve hot.

<u>**Serves 4**</u>. One serving is about 225 Calories.

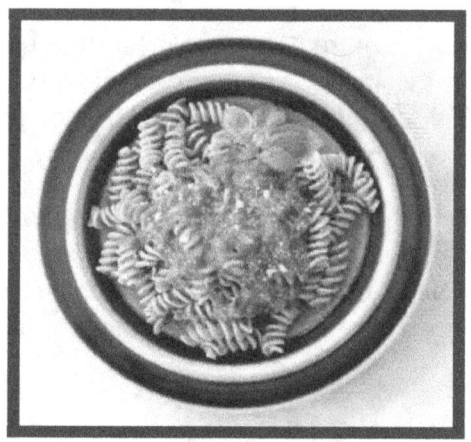

<u>**Diet Tip of the Day:**</u> **Beware of alcoholic beverages**. Beer has about 13 Calories per ounce, wine 25 Calories per ounce and whiskey 71 Calories per ounce.

Day 14a - Recipe

Low-Cal Smoothie

Smoothies are delicious, nutritious and fun to drink! They're great for a fast but nutritious breakfast, a light energy-boosting lunch, a healthy snack, a late afternoon pick me up, and a delicious dessert. Making your own smoothie is a smart way to save money and get healthy at the same time!

  8 ounces plain fat-free yogurt
  1 cup orange juice
  1 cup strawberries
  ½ cup blueberries
  1 banana
  1 teaspoon sugar
  1 teaspoon vanilla extract

Place yogurt, strawberries, and blueberries in a blender. Pour in orange juice. Add sugar and vanilla extract to mixture. Blend all ingredients until thick and smooth. Pour smoothie into a glass and enjoy.

Serves 2. About 220 Calories per serving

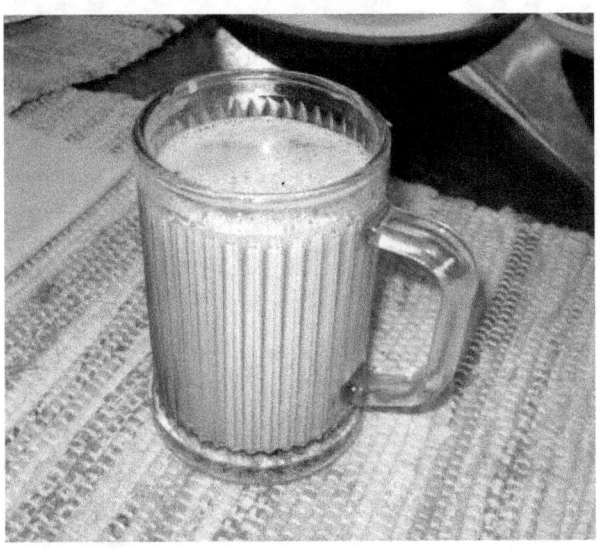

Day 14b - Recipe

Frozen-Fish Dinner

No recipe today. No cooking today. It's your day off! Some reasonably good frozen fish dinners are:
- Lean Cuisine Shrimp Alfredo (200 Cal)
- Lean Cuisine Parmesan Crusted Fish (290 Cal)
- Lean Cuisine Salmon with Basil (250 Cal)
- Healthy Choice Herb-Crusted Fish (270 Cal)

That's it. At this writing, there are just not that many frozen fish dinners for sale at supermarkets, although new entrees are being introduced continually. If you choose any of the above entrees, you will not use all of the **300 Calories allocated for this meal**. In this case, use the excess 100 or so calories anyway you wish. Splurge on extra dessert or save the calories for another day!

Please read the important **Frozen-Food Safety Warning** in **Appendix C page 117**.

Diet Tip of the Day: Two scientific journals indicate **dark chocolate** - not white chocolate or milk chocolate - is potent antioxidant and is good for you. But don't overdo it, because you have to offset the extra chocolate calories by eating less of other foods.

Day 15 Recipe

Vegetables with Couscous

1 10-ounce box couscous
1 red bell pepper, cut into strips
1 yellow bell pepper, cut into strips
1 small yellow squash, sliced
1 small zucchini, sliced
1 teaspoon salt
¾ teaspoon black pepper
¾ teaspoon minced garlic
¾ teaspoon Italian seasoning
2 tablespoon olive oil
3 tablespoon balsamic vinegar
5 ounces feta cheese

1. Pre-heat oven to 425 °F.
2. Prepare couscous according to package directions.
3. In a small bowl, whisk together marinade of salt, pepper, garlic, Italian seasoning, olive oil and balsamic vinegar and toss with pepper strips, sliced squash and zucchini.
4. Spread vegetables evenly in sheet pan and roast for 10 to 12 minutes or until vegetables are crisp-tender. Reserve left over marinade.
5. Allow vegetables to cool slightly, then toss with remaining marinade, couscous and feta cheese.

Serves 6. About 330 Calories per serving

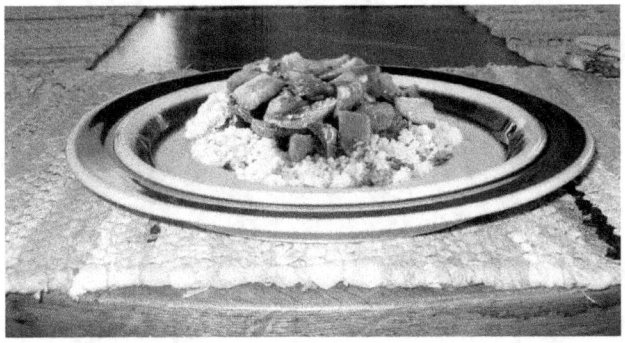

Diet Tip of the Day: **Stay Busy.** Most people will do anything to avoid work, housework, yard work, exercise, etc. But any kind of work burns a lot more calories than sitting! Whatever it is you are avoiding – go do it!

Day 16 Recipe
Baked Red Snapper
4 red snapper fillets – 4 oz each
(salmon may be substituted)
½ cup white wine
½ cup non-fat yogurt mixed with half as much mustard
½ pound green beans
20 cherry tomatoes
4 tsp olive oil
1 cup wild rice, brown rice and grain berry mix

Prepare rice mix per package directions.

Brown fillets in non-stick pan. Place fillets skin side down in baking dish coated with non-stick spray. Add white wine and cook in oven preheated to 350 ºF for about 15 minutes. Spoon pan juices over fillets. Salt and pepper to taste.

Place green beans in skillet. Add ¼-inch of water and cook over medium heat until water boils off. Add cherry tomatoes and olive oil. Stir well and sauté for a few minutes. Season with fresh rosemary and oregano. Salt and pepper to taste.

Plate red snapper fillet and spoon over yogurt-mustard sauce. Add green beans & tomato mix and the wild rice. Serve hot.

Serves 4. One plate consisting of one snapper fillet (215 Calories) with green beans & tomato mix (75 Calories) and wild rice (160 Calories) totals 450 Calories.

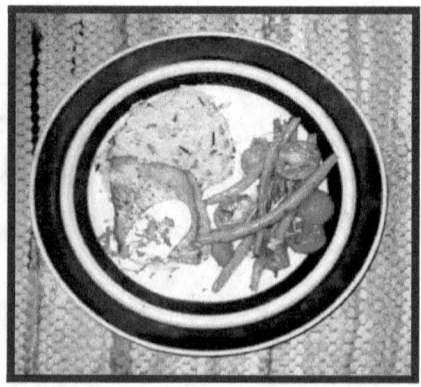

Diet Tip of the Day: **Don't have sweets in your house**. This makes them easier to resist. Out of sight, out of mind!

Day 17 Recipe

Tofu-Veggie Stir Fry

Citrus Sauce:
- 6 tablespoons cooking wine
- ¼ cup orange juice
- 1 tablespoon light soy sauce
- 2 teaspoons toasted sesame oil
- 1 teaspoon grated or minced fresh ginger
- 1 teaspoon cornstarch
- 1 tablespoon toasted sesame seeds

Stir Fry:
- 1 (14-ounce) package firm tofu, drained
- 1 tablespoon cooking oil
- 1½ cups fresh or frozen sugar snap peas
- 3 medium carrots, thinly sliced
- ¾ cup thinly sliced onion

1. Stir together sauce ingredients. Set aside while preparing stir fry.
2. Press and pat tofu dry with a towel to remove excess water. Cut into ½-inch cubes.
3. Heat a large skillet or wok over medium-high heat. Add oil and tofu; stir frequently until tofu is lightly browned, about 5 minutes. Add snow peas, carrots and onion. Stir-fry about 5 minutes until vegetables are cooked, but still crisp.
4. Stir in prepared sauce and cook 1-2 minutes until sauce is slightly thickened. Serve immediately.

<u>**Serves 4.**</u> 230 Calories per serving

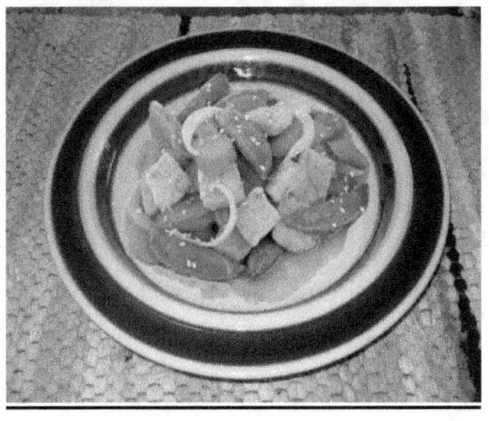

Day 18 Recipe

Grilled Swordfish

1¼ pounds swordfish
1 bottle citrus-herb marinade
24 cherry tomatoes
4 medium potatoes
2 cups fresh spinach
1 tsp rosemary & juice of ¼ lemon
2 tsp extra virgin olive oil (Evoo)

Steam spinach with garlic and drizzle with Evoo. Cut up potatoes and place sprinkle with lemon juice, add rosemary, salt and black pepper. Place on grill for about 10 minutes, turning occasionally.

Toss cherry tomatoes in small amount Evoo. Add fresh oregano, salt and black pepper. Place on heavy-duty aluminum foil, seal and grill for about 3 minutes.

Marinade swordfish in citrus-herb vinaigrette. Grill on hot fire for about 5 minutes on one side and 3 minutes on the other, or until done as desired.

Serves 4. One plate consisting of grilled swordfish (250 Calories) with grilled potatoes (100 Calories) and cherry tomatoes (45 Calories) and steamed spinach (50 Calories) totals 445 Calories.

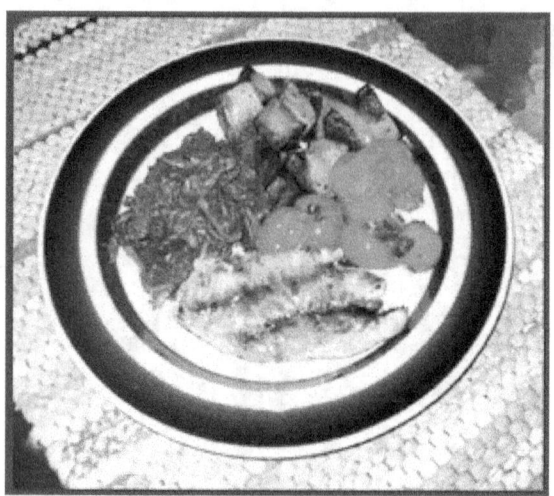

Diet Tip of the Day: Don't be in a hurry to lose weight. Slow weight loss is healthier, is more likely to be permanent, and is easier to sustain over the long haul.

Day 19 Recipe

Vegetarian Dinner - Out

No recipe today. No cooking today. Have dinner at your favorite vegetarian restaurant, but make sure you choose a restaurant where you have a fighting chance to achieve your calorie goal. For your vegetarian dinner out, your maximum allowable calories (including appetizer, soup, main course and dessert) are as follows:
- For the **1200 Calorie Diet**: 530 Calories
- For the **1500 Calorie Diet**: 630 Calories

Tips for Eating Vegetarian Out: First, order simple such as tofu stir fried with vegetables, and brown rice. Tell the waiter you want little to no added sauce or gravy. Estimate the calories in the meal: tofu is about 75 Calories per ounce, most vegetable servings average approximately 50 Calories per cup, rice is about 100 Calories per ½ cup, and add about 150 Calories for the oil used in the stir fry. Then knowing your allowable calorie total for the meal, decide how much to eat – and take the remainder home. If fresh fruit is not an option, pass on dessert and have the evening snack specified for that day on this diet.

In a restaurant, most nutritionists recommend you eat the low-calorie items on your plate first. Start with the salad, soup and veggies. By the time you get to the legumes and starches you will hopefully be full enough to be content with smaller portions of the higher-calorie choices.

Incidentally, if you live in a small town with no vegetarian restaurant, to stay on this diet, have a frozen vegetarian entree. And try to abide by the allowable calorie total.

Finally, some dieticians advise their dieting clients not to eat out. That's right. They believe eating at home is safer. But our thought is you have to eat out eventually so why not learn how while your resolve is high?

Diet Tip of the Day: Another dilemma for dieters is **judging portion size**. It makes no sense to worry about whether to apportion 70 or 80 Calories per ounce for a cut of lean meat if you have no idea whether the portion you are planning to eat weighs four or ten ounces. To be successful, you must learn to estimate portion sizes with reasonable accuracy.

Day 20 Recipe
Quick Pasta alla Puttanesca
This famous pasta dish originated in Naples. Puttanesca means "ladies of the night." The exact origin of the name is unclear, but one thing is clear: It's delicious! Here is one of many recipe versions.

½ pound spaghetti (whole grain preferred)
20 black pitted olives
1 can (14½ oz) diced tomatoes
½ can (4 oz) tomato sauce
2 Tbsp Evoo
3 cloves of garlic, chopped and 1Tbsp dried minced onion
½ tsp crushed red pepper flakes
1 Tbsp capers drained and rinsed
¼ cup currants

Cook spaghetti according to package directions. Drain and return spaghetti to pot; add a teaspoon Evoo and toss to coat.
Heat 2 tablespoons olive oil in large skillet over medium-high heat. Add red pepper flakes; cook and stir 1 to 2 minutes or until sizzling. Add onion and garlic; cook and stir 1 minute. Finally, add tomatoes with juice, tomato sauce, olives, currants and capers. Cook over medium-high heat, stirring frequently, until sauce is heated through.
Serves 4. About 345 Calories per serving

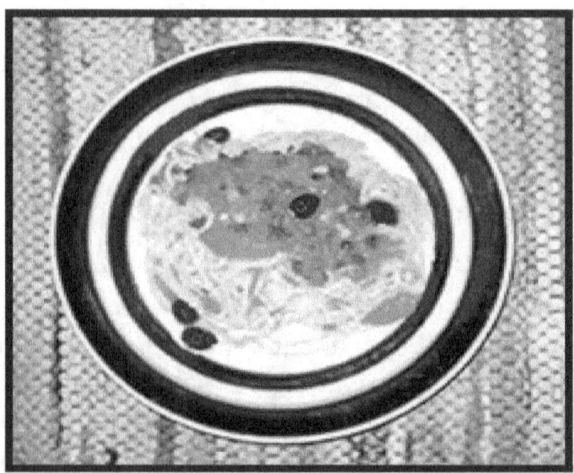

Diet Tip of the Day: Dilute juices, such as apple juice, orange, etc. with water. This cuts the flavor slightly but really reduces calorie content.

Day 21 Recipe
Frozen-Pasta Dinner
No recipe today. No cooking today. It's your day off! Some reasonably good frozen pasta dinners are:
- Lean Cuisine Angel Hair Pomodoro (220 Cal)
- Lean Cuisine Cheese Ravioli (250 Cal)
- Healthy Choice Portobella Spinach Parmesan (230 Cal)
- Healthy Choice Portobella Marsala Pasta (230 Cal)
- Amy's Light & Lean Spagehetti Italiano (240 Cal)

If you choose any of the above entrees, you will not use all of the **300 Calories allocated for this meal**. In this case, use the excess 100 or so calories anyway you wish. Splurge on extra dessert or save the calories for another day!

Please read the important **Frozen-Food Safety Warning** in **Appendix C, page 117.**

Diet Tip of the Day: A good understanding of nutrition is not only vital for good health but also will help you control your weight over the long term. For example, did you know that foods that are an "excellent source" of a particular nutrient provide 20% or more of the Recommended Daily Value. Whereas, foods that are a "good source" of a nutrient provide between 10 and 20% of the Recommended Daily Value.

Day 22 Recipe

Tomato Risotto Salad

1 bag microwave-in-bag green beans
1¾ cups lower-sodium vegetable broth
2 tablespoons butter
1 small onion
2 cups Arborio rice
2 pounds ripe tomatoes
2 cups fresh corn kernels
2 ounces grated Parmesan cheese
2 tablespoons chopped basil

1) Cook green beans according to package directions. Cut into 1-inch. pieces.

2) In 2-quart saucepan, heat broth and 2 cups water to boiling. While broth mixture heats, in 4-quart bowl, microwave butter and onion, uncovered, on high for 3 minutes or until softened. Stir in rice and cook another minute.

3) Stir broth-water mixture into rice mixture. Cover with vented plastic wrap; microwave on medium (50% power) about 10 minutes.

4) Meanwhile, in food processor, puree half of tomatoes; strain juice through sieve into measuring cup, pressing on solids. Discard solids and chop remaining tomatoes. Stir 1½cups tomato juice into rice mixture. Cover with vented plastic wrap and microwave on Medium heat 5 minutes or until liquid is absorbed.

5) Stir corn into rice mixture. Cover with vented plastic wrap; microwave on Medium 3 minutes or until corn is heated through. Stir Parmesan cheese, green beans, tomatoes, half of basil, ½ teaspoon salt, and ¼ teaspoon pepper into rice mixture (the risotto). Sprinkle with basil.
Serves 6. 370 Calories per serving.

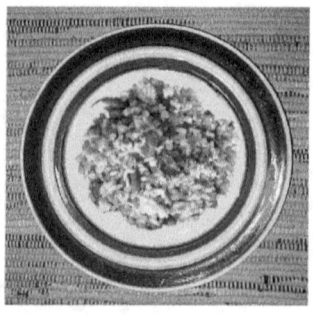

Day 23 Recipe

Beans & Greens Salad

⅓ cup chopped oregano
⅓ cup chopped parsley
3 cloves garlic, chopped
1 lemon, juiced

Prepare salad dressing by combining above ingredients and stirring in ¼ cup Evoo. Salt and pepper to taste.

½ pound mesclun mix
¼ pound green beans
1 19 oz can garbanzo beans (chickpeas)

Arrange mesclun mix, garbanzo beans and green beans on a large platter. Drizzle salad dressing over beans and greens.

Serves 4. Approximately 260 Calories per serving.

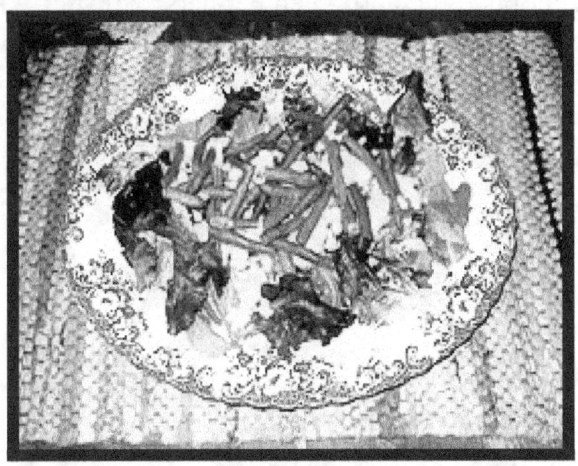

Diet Tip of the Day: Beans are a wonderful food but they are an incomplete protein. If however beans are eaten with a whole-grain bread, the combination forms a complete protein – just as complete and nutritious as meat, poultry, or fish.

Day 24 Recipe
Four-Bean Plus Salad
Note that the total caloric value of the salad will change very little, if the proportions of the bean varieties and corn are varied – according to taste.

½ cup canned red kidney beans, drained and rinsed
½ cup canned black beans, drained and rinsed
½ cup canned chick peas, drained and rinsed
½ cup canned cannelloni beans, drained and rinsed
½ cup canned corn, drained
1 small red pepper, chopped
1 small green pepper, chopped
2 Tbsp Evoo
2 Tbsp lemon juice

In a large bowl mix red kidney beans, black beans, chick peas, cannelloni beans, corn and chopped red and green peppers. Stir in Evoo and lemon juice and plate.

Serves about 6. One serving is ½ cup – with about 135 Calories

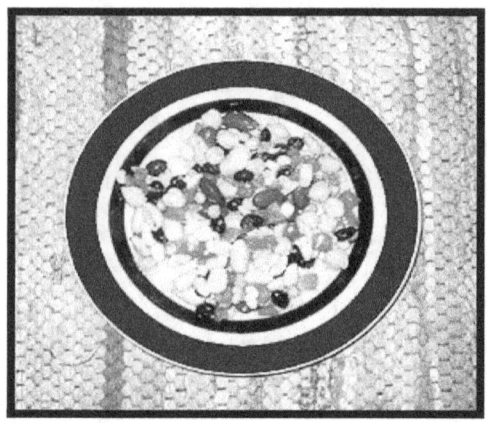

Note: Reserve 1 cup for lunch on Day 27.

Diet Tip of the Day: Vigorous exercise doesn't necessarily stimulate you to overeat. Just the opposite. In many cases, exercise actually helps curb your appetite – immediately following a workout.

Day 25 - Recipe

Tofu with Veggies & Peanuts

2 3½-ounce bags boil-in-bag jasmine rice
1 14-ounce package water-packed firm tofu
½ cup fat-free, less-sodium vegetable broth
1 tablespoon ground fresh chili paste
1 tablespoon less-sodium soy sauce
1 teaspoon cornstarch
2 teaspoons black bean garlic sauce
1 tablespoon canola oil
1 8-ounce package pre-sliced mushrooms
1 tablespoon bottled ground fresh ginger
¼ teaspoon salt
½ cup matchstick-cut carrots
½ cup chopped green onions
¼ cup unsalted dry-roasted peanuts, chopped

1. Preheat broiler. Cook rice according to package directions, omitting salt and fat.
2. Drain tofu and cut into 1-inch pieces. (For tofu draining and preparation tips go to page 113.) Arrange tofu in a single layer on a foil-lined pan coated with cooking spray. Broil 14 minutes or until golden.
3. While tofu cooks, combine broth and next 4 ingredients (through black bean sauce), stirring with a whisk; set aside.
4. Heat oil in a large nonstick skillet over medium-high heat. Add salt and mushrooms; sauté 4 minutes or until mushrooms begin to release liquid, stirring occasionally. Stir in carrots and ginger; cook 1 minute. Add broth mixture; cook 30 seconds or until sauce begins to thicken. Remove from heat; stir in tofu and onions. Serve over rice; sprinkle with peanuts.
Serves 4. About 320 Calories per serving

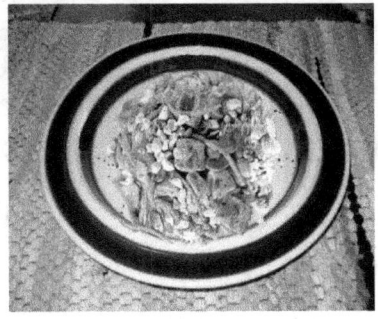

Day 26 Recipe

Grilled Scallops and Polenta

1 pound sea scallops
¾ cup polenta cornmeal
¾ cup skim milk
1 medium Portobello mushroom
½ pound green beans
¼ cup chopped red onion
16 asparagus spear
1 tsp Evoo

Bring 1½ cups of water and skim milk to rapid boil. Add salt to taste and slowly add polenta while stirring. Reduce heat. Continue stirring until desired consistency is reached. Pour polenta into lightly greased pan. After polenta has cooled cover and refrigerate. Cut chilled polenta into 4 pieces. Grill on medium-hot fire – about two minutes on each side. Brush Portobello mushroom and asparagus spear with Evoo and place on grill for about 3 minutes on each side.
Grill scallops on medium-hot fire. Turn after two minutes or when first side turns opaque. Grill until second side turns opaque – about another 2 minutes. Don't overcook but test a scallop by cutting to make sure it's cooked through. Salt and pepper to taste.
Serves 4. The food on the plate pictured below totals 380 Calories.

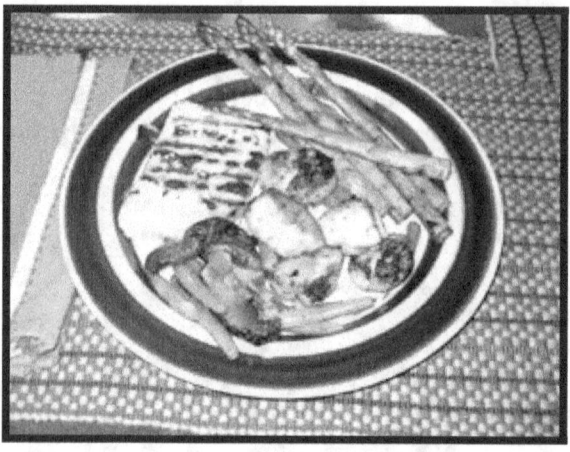

Diet Tip of the Day: To have better control of what you eat **bring your lunch to work**.

Day 27 Recipe
Fettuccine in Summer Sauce
This sauce is often served in the summer because it's lighter than what is usually dished up with pasta. But despite its name the sauce is wonderful year round.

½ pound fettuccine
8 ounces fresh asparagus, trimmed & cut into 2" pieces
20 cherry tomatoes, halved
2 Tbsp plus 1 tsp Evoo
2 cloves of garlic, chopped
½ small onion, diced

Cook fettuccine according to package directions. Drain and return pasta to pot; add a teaspoon Evoo and toss to coat. Meanwhile steam asparagus and drain.
In large skillet over medium-high heat, sauté cherry tomatoes in 2 Tbsp olive oil until skin begins to crack. Add onion and cook until translucent. Stir in garlic . Thin sauce with pasta liquid to desired consistency. Toss cooked pasta and asparagus into sauce and serve immediately.
Serves 4. About 290 Calories per serving

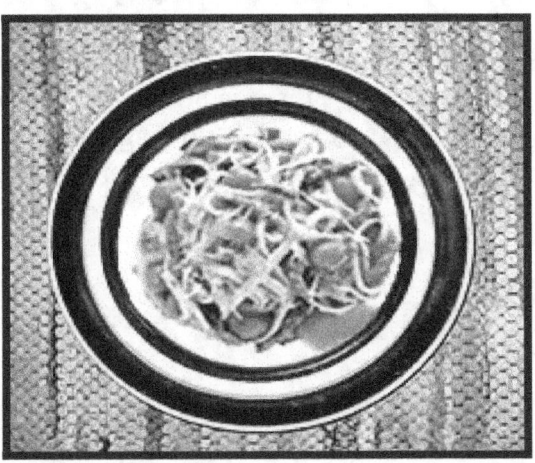

Diet Tip of the Day: A major weight-loss fallacy is that you can get rid of abdominal fat by working your abdominal muscles. This is based on the incorrect belief that fat is eliminated from a particular part of your body if you engage the muscles underneath that layer of fat. No such luck.

Day 28 Recipe
Frozen Vegetarian Meal

No recipe today. No cooking today. It's your day off! Some reasonably good frozen vegetarian dinners are:
- Amy's Indian Vegetable Korma (310 Cal)
- Amy's Thai Stir Fry (310 Cal)
- Amy's Asian Noodle Stir Fry (300 Cal)
- Lean Cuisine Veggie Scramble (180 Cal)
- Lean Cuisine Mushroom & Spring Pea Risotto (240 Cal)
- Healthy Choice Asian Potstickers (330 Cal)

Note that if you choose any of the above entrees, you will not use all of the **340 Calories allocated for this meal**. In this case, use the excess 100 or so calories anyway you wish. Splurge on extra dessert or save the calories for another day!

Please read the important **Frozen-Food Safety Warning** in **Appendix C,** page 117.

<u>Diet Tip of the Day:</u>   The **general weight-change rule is "last on first off."** Assume as you gained weight, the first place you noticed it was on your thighs, next your buttocks, then your face. As you lose weight, it generally will come off in the reverse order, first from your face, then your rear and finally your thighs. And there is not much you can do about that. The truth is there is no food, no exercise, no magic belt, and no pill that will cause your body to lose fat in one place rather than another.

Day 29 Recipe

Barbequed Shrimp

1½ pounds large shrimp
3 Tbsp bottled barbeque sauce
4 medium ears of corn

Pour barbeque sauce into shallow bowl. Toss shrimp in barbeque sauce to coat. Place shrimp on medium-hot grill. Turn shrimp after about two minutes or when shrimp turn pink. Grill until second side turns pink – approximately another 2 minutes. Don't overcook but test a shrimp by cutting to make sure it is cooked through. Salt and pepper to taste. Serve hot or at room temperature.

Serves 4. About 160 Calories per serving (shrimp only).

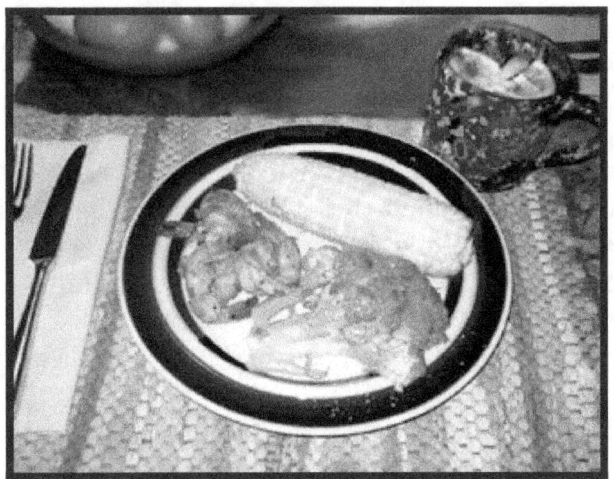

Diet Tip of the Day: A very important weight-profile parameter is your waist-to-hip ratio. Health risks for heart attack and stroke increase considerably for men with a ratio above 1.0 and for women with a ratio above 0.8. To calculate your ratio, measure your waist size (at its narrowest circumference) and divide it by your hip size (at the widest section).

Day 30 Recipe
Tofu Steak with Veggies

⅓ cup white miso (soybean paste)
⅓ cup mirin (sweet rice wine)
⅓ cup rice vinegar
1 tablespoon finely grated peeled fresh ginger
½ cup chopped dry-roasted peanuts, divided
5 tablespoons sesame oil, divided
2 (14-ounce) packages water-packed firm tofu, drained
8 cups salad greens

1. Combine white miso, mirin, ¼ cup peanuts, and 3 tablespoons oil in a small bowl; stir with a whisk.
2. Cut each tofu block crosswise into 8 (½-inch-thick) slices. Arrange tofu on several layers of paper towels. Top with several more layers of paper towels; top with a cast-iron skillet or other heavy pan. Let stand 30 minutes. Remove tofu from paper towels.
3. Heat 1 tablespoon oil in a large nonstick skillet over medium-high heat. Add 4 tofu slices to pan; sauté 4 minutes on each side or until crisp and golden. Remove from pan, and drain tofu on paper towels. Repeat procedure with remaining 1 tablespoon oil and remaining 4 tofu slices.
4. Place 1 cup greens on each of 8 plates. Top each serving with 2 tofu slices, 3 tablespoons miso mixture, and 1½ teaspoons chopped peanuts.

<u>Serves 8</u>: About 275 Calories per serving.

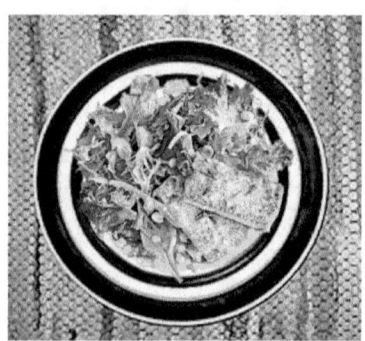

<u>Diet Tip of the Day:</u> Plan to be on a diet the rest of your life. Not necessarily a weight reducing diet. At some point you'll want to just maintain your weight. But you will still need to continue to make good healthy food choices – and not slip back to your old eating habits.

Appendix A
Vegetarian
Background & Nutrition

People choose a vegetarian, or plant-based diet, for reasons based on nutrition, health, taste, morality, religion, culture, ethics, aesthetics, environment, economy, or politics.

Vegetarian Benefits

Compared to meat eaters, vegetarians have a lower overall mortality rate and a reduced incidence of heart disease, type 2 diabetes and stroke. And a vegetarian diet has been shown to reduce the risk of some cancers.

Properly planned vegetarian diets have been found to satisfy nutritional needs for all stages of life. Such diets have lower levels of saturated fat and cholesterol and higher levels of carbohydrates, fiber, magnesium, potassium, folate and antioxidants such as vitamins C and E and phytochemicals. And most nutritionists agree that properly planned vegetarian diets are nutritionally adequate and provide health benefits in the prevention and treatment of certain diseases. Large-scale studies have shown vegetarian diets significantly lower the risk of colon cancer, heart disease, high blood pressure and other diseases. In fact, many health-care professionals think that eating a healthy vegetarian diet is one of the best things you can do for your short-term and long-term health. In fact, a well planned vegetarian diet provides the same level of nutrients as a meat-eater's diet.

On the other hand, poorly planned vegetarian diets can increase the risk of cardiovascular disease, blood clots and platelet disorders. (These risks can be offset by sufficient consumption of vitamin B_{12} and polyunsaturated fatty acids.)

Vegetarian Nutrition

Vegetarian, or not, you should always consider the health effects of what you eat. Be sure to replace meat with healthy foods and eat a balanced diet. Eat a variety of whole grains, vegetables and protein foods, such as tofu or veggie burgers to stay full and healthy. While eating an adequate amount of protein is important for vegetarians, getting sufficient calcium and iron (and if you are a vegan vitamin B_{12}) are equally important.

The problem with some vegetarian diets is that they are often relatively low in omega-3 fatty acids and vitamin B_{12}. Conversely, high levels of dietary fiber, folic acid, vitamins C and E, and magnesium, and low consumption of saturated fat are all beneficial aspects of a vegetarian diet.

A well-balanced vegetarian diet with plenty of whole grains, fruits and vegetables is one of the healthiest diets on the planet. You do, however, need to make sure you get ample amounts of the following vital nutrients and micronutrients.

Protein
Most people eat too much protein – not too little of it. Adults need about 0.79 grams of protein for every kilogram of body weight per day to keep from slowly breaking down their own tissue. (That translates as approximately 0.36 grams of protein for every pound of body weight.) A case in point, an adult female weighing 154 pounds (70 kg) requires about (154 x 0.36), or 55 grams of protein per day. An adult male weighing 180 pounds requires (180 x 0.36), or 65 grams per day. How much protein is in food? A few examples: There are approximately seven grams of protein per ounce of beef, poultry, fish, cheese or peanuts. Soybeans pack 10 grams of protein per ounce. Most other beans and lentils contain about six grams of protein per ounce. There are roughly three grams of protein in an ounce of whole-grain cereal, and milk has one gram of protein per fluid ounce.

One cup of tofu contains about 20 grams of protein. Lots of foods contain protein and if vegetarians eat a well-balanced diet, they should undoubtedly consume more than enough protein without even thinking about it. Lacto-ovo vegetarians get sufficient protein from eggs and dairy. Pescaterians get all the protein they need from sea food, eggs and dairy. While vegans can get their protein from tofu, veggie burgers, soy, lentils, chickpeas, nuts and seeds, brown rice and whole grains.

Proteins are composed of amino acids. Often a concern with vegetarian and non-vegetarian is adequate intake of the eight essential amino acids, which cannot be synthesized by humans. While dairy and egg products provide complete protein sources for ovo-lacto vegetarians, several vegetable foods such as, soy, lupin beans, pumpkin seeds, hempseed, chia seeds, amaranth, buckwheat, pistachio nuts, and quinoa, also have significant amounts of all eight types of essential amino acids.

Essential amino acids, can also be obtained by eating complementary plant sources that, in combination, provide all eight essential amino acids (e.g. brown rice and beans, whole wheat pasta and beans, or hummus and whole wheat pita,- though combining these in the same meal is not necessary). Protein intake in vegetarian diets is often lower than in meat diets but usually meets the daily requirements of most people. Numerous studies confirm that vegetarian diets supply sufficient protein provided a variety of plant sources are consumed.

Iron

Vegetarian diets typically contain similar levels of iron to non-vegetarian diets, but the iron is often not absorbed as well as iron from meat sources. In addition, iron absorption is sometimes inhibited by other foods in the diet. Some dieticians recommend consuming foods high in vitamin C, such as citrus fruit or juices, tomatoes, or broccoli, as a way to increase the amount of iron absorbed. Vegetarian foods that are rich in iron are black beans, kidney beans, broccoli, lentils, oatmeal, raisins, spinach, cabbage, lettuce, black-eyed peas, soybeans, many breakfast cereals, sunflower seeds, chickpeas, tomato juice, molasses, thyme, and whole-wheat bread. Vegan diets are often higher in iron than lacto-vegetarian diets, because dairy products are low in iron. The American Dietetic Association, asserts that iron deficiency is no more common in vegetarians than in meat eaters, and iron deficiency anemia is rare in all diets.

Vitamin B_{12}

Vitamin B_{12} is not generally found in plants but is occurs naturally in foods of animal origin. Lacto-ovo vegetarians can obtain vitamin B_{12} from dairy products and eggs, while vegans can obtain vitamin B_{12} from a dietary supplement and fortified foods (such as some soy products and breakfast cereals). The recommended dietary allowance for B_{12} in the United States is 2.4 mcg per day and 2.8 mcg per day for lactating females. Although the daily requirement for vitamin B_{12} is very small, a vitamin B_{12} deficiency is very serious and can lead to anemia and irreversible nerve damage.

Fatty Acids

Omega-3 and omega-6 fatty acids are called "essential" fats for good reason. Humans need them for many functions, from building healthy cells to maintaining brain and nerve function. But our bodies cannot produce them. The only source is food. These polyunsaturated fats are also important because they lower the risk of heart disease. Some studies suggest these fats may also protect against type 2 diabetes, Alzheimer's disease, and age-related brain decline.

Omega-6 comes from soybean oil, corn oil and sunflower oil, as well as from nuts and seeds. The American Heart Association recommends that at least 5% to 10% of daily food calories come from omega-6 fatty acids. Omega-3 comes primarily from fatty fish such as salmon, mackerel, and tuna, and in lesser amounts from walnuts and flaxseeds.

Calcium

Calcium intake in vegetarians and vegans can be similar to that in meat eaters, provided the diet is properly planned. Lacto-ovo vegetarians consume dairy products and can obtain calcium from dairy sources like milk, yogurt, and cheese. Non-dairy milks that are fortified with calcium, such as soymilk and almond milk also contribute a significant amount of calcium to the diet. The calcium found in broccoli, bok choy, and kale is also well absorbed by the body. Though the calcium content per serving is lower in these vegetables than in a glass of milk, the absorption of the calcium is higher. Other foods that contain calcium include calcium-set tofu, blackstrap molasses, turnip greens, mustard greens, soybeans, almonds, okra, and dried figs. Although calcium is found in spinach, Swiss chard, beans and beet greens, the calcium in these foods is poorly absorbed by humans.

Vitamin D

Vitamin D is found in many foods, including fish, eggs, fortified milk, and cod liver oil. In addition, 10 minutes of sensible daily sun exposure is sufficient to prevent vitamin D deficiency. Vitamin D comes in several different types. Two forms are important to humans: vitamin D2, which is made by plants, and vitamin D3, which is made by human skin when exposed to sunlight. Foods may also be fortified with vitamin D2 or D3. The major role of vitamin D is to maintain normal blood levels of calcium and phosphorus. Vitamin D helps the body absorb calcium, which forms and maintains strong bones. It is used alone or together with calcium to improve bone health and decrease fractures. Vitamin D is thought to also protect against osteoporosis, high blood pressure, cancer, and other diseases.

Tofu Info

Tofu is an excellent non-animal high-protein food made from soybeans that is frequently linked with vegetarianism. Tofu comes in two basic varieties: soft or silken tofu and firm or regular tofu. Tofu has no taste but readily absorbs the flavor of other foods. Refrigerate tofu after you open a package and use it within four days.

Tofu can help you lose weight. Half-cup of **tofu** contains only about 90 calories, whereas the same amount of other proteins such as ground beef which contains 331 calories and cheese which has 320 calories

Firm versions of tofu (well-drained) are used for kebabs, mock meats, and dishes requiring a consistency that holds together, while the softer tofu styles are used in desserts, soups, shakes, and sauces. Grated firm western tofu is sometimes used as a meat substitute and can be barbecued because it will hold together on a barbecue grill. Soft tofu is sometimes used as a dairy-free or low-calorie filler. Silken tofu may be used to replace cheese in certain dishes such as lasagna.

Most proteins are delicious even when seasoned simply with salt and pepper. Not tofu which most often tofu tastes bland. But you can turn it into a food you actually want to eat with the following tips.

Buying Tofu

Tofu is usually found in a refrigerated case in the produce department (fruit and vegetables) of most supermarkets. Some stores have tofu in the dairy section and others in stock it in health-food.

Preparing Tofu

1) Most tofu comes packed in water. But a water-logged block of tofu won't absorb a marinade or get crispy in a frying pan. The first thing to do is drain the block as much as possible. To drain it, slice the block and place the slices on a paper towel-lined baking sheet. Top tofu with more paper towels and then a heavy object. Let tofu sit at least one hour. Once drained, you can marinate the tofu or start cooking it.

2) After pressing, tofu is ready to absorb flavor. But the tofu still retains some water and oil and water don't mix. In most cases, use soy, citrus, or vinegar-based marinades instead.

3) Trying to get tofu crispy is difficult. Tossing tofu in cornstarch overcomes the difficulty. Place cornstarch in a bowl, add drained or marinated tofu pieces, and toss. A light coating is best.

4) To sear tofu, use sesame oil which can take the heat and doubles as a flavoring agent, giving the tofu a nutty flavor.

Leftover Tofu

Once a package of tofu is opened it will last about three days if refrigerated. You can freeze leftover tofu. Frozen tofu can last up to three months. And you can freeze any kind of tofu: silken, firm, or extra-firm. Just cut the tofu into cubes and freeze the cubes on a baking sheet. Once hard, store the tofu together in a freezer container. Thaw leftover tofu on a counter top during dinner prep. Thawed tofu can be cooked just as fresh tofu. But squeeze the tofu gently before cooking to eliminate extra moisture.

Appendix B
Vegetarian Soup

The following lists soup selections that come in cans and microwavable bowls. See the important note at the end of list regarding serving size. Valid as of 07/30/20.

Soup Description	Container	Calories
Amy's Organic Chunky Vegetable	Canned	60
Amy's Organic Minestrone	Canned	90
Healthy Choice Cheese Tortellini	Microwaveable	90
Amy's Organic Split Pea	Canned	100
Amy's No Chicken Noodle	Canned	100
Amy's Organic Butternut Squash	Canned	100
Healthy Choice Country Vegetable	Microwaveable	100
Amy's Organic Vegan Chunky Tomato	Canned	110
Healthy Choice Red Bean and Rice	Microwaveable	130
Healthy Choice Tomato Basil	Microwaveable	130
Amy's Organic Southwestern Vegetable	Canned	140
Amy's Organic Hearty Spanish Rice &	Canned	140
Amy's Organic Hearty Rustic Italian	Canned	140
Amy's Organic Thai Coconut	Canned	140
Healthy Choice Vegetable Barley	Microwaveable	140
Amy's Organic Quinoa, Kale & Red	Canned	150
Healthy Choice Traditional Lentil	Microwaveable	160
Amy's Organic Lentil Vegetable	Canned	160
Amy's Indian Golden Lentil	Canned	220

* **Important:** When the Daily Meal Plan menu specifies soup, have only one serving (usually this is 1 cup = 8 ounces) unless stated otherwise.

APPENDIX C
Frozen Food Safety

Increasingly, food giants like ConAgra, Nestlé and others that supply Americans with processed foods concede that they cannot ensure the safety of their food products. Frozen foods pose a particularly serious safety problem because unsuspecting consumers buy frozen foods for their convenience and incorrectly believe that cooking frozen foods is a matter of taste – not safety.

Still the food industry says that extensive outbreaks of food-borne illness are rare, even though it is well-known that most of the millions of cases of food-borne illness every year go unreported or are not traced to the source. For example, each year approximately 40,000 cases of salmonella poisoning are reported in the United States – but perhaps as many as one million cases go unreported. (Salmonella is a type of bacteria most often found in poultry, eggs, unprocessed milk, meat and water.) Recently salmonella pathogens in some frozen meals have sickened thousands of people.

How could this happen? First, the supply chain for ingredients in processed foods – from flour to fruits and vegetables to flavorings – is becoming more complex and global in the drive to keep food costs down. As a result, government and industry officials concede that almost every food ingredient is now a potential carrier of pathogens. A further complication is that a large number of food companies subcontract processing work to save money and don't require suppliers to test for pathogens. In fact, companies often don't even know who is supplying their ingredients.

In addition, many frozen-food manufacturers have stopped cooking their products at high temperatures, a tactic they call the "kill step," which is intended to eliminate any lingering microbes. Frequently this process step turns some of the frozen food ingredients into mush. So, instead the "kill step" has been shifted to consumers. For example, ConAgra has added food safety instructions to its frozen meals, including the Healthy Choice brand. A typical "frozen-food safety" instruction offers this guidance: "Internal temperature needs to reach 165°F as measured by a food thermometer in several spots."

Moreover, General Mills, now advises consumers to avoid microwaves altogether and cook their frozen pizzas only in a conventional oven.

Bottom line: To be safe, always cook frozen foods so that the internal temperature reaches 165°F as measured by a good food thermometer.

APPENDIX D
Calories in Foods

Zero Calorie Foods
Beverages
Coffee without added sugar, cream, or milk
Tea without added sugar, cream, or milk
Carbonated beverages, artificially sweetened
Diet soda
Seltzer water, Sparkling water
Seasoning Agents
Celery seasoning*, Celery salt
Chives seasoning*
Cinnamon
Curry powder
Dill, Garlic*
Herbs, Horseradish*
Lemon juice, sections, or slices*
Lime juice, sections, or slices*
Mint
Monosodium glutamate
Mustard, Onion salt
Onion seasoning*
Paprika, Parsley*
Pepper, all varieties
Peppers, garden, red or green, as seasoning*
Pimiento as seasoning*
Salt, Salt substitutes
Sauces (Worcestershire, A-1, Tabasco
Spices
Vinegar, cider, or wine
Relishes
Bread and butter pickles*
Cucumber & Dill pickles*
India relish*
Pickled onion*
Sour pickles*

Soups
Bouillon
Clear soups without fat
Consommé*
Jellied clear soups*
Jellied consommé*
Tomato bouillon*
Jellied madrilène*
Others
Gelatin, unsweetened*
Sugar Substitutes
Saccharin, Aspartame
* These items contain a few calories, but the calorie counts are negligible when they are used as seasoning, a relish or a thickening agent.

Calories in Beverages
Soda such as Colas, 7-Up (8 oz) ..100 Calories
Beer & ale (12 oz) ....175 Calories
Dry wines (4 oz) ....100 Calories
Whisky (jigger) ....125 Calories
Cocktail (12 oz) .... 150 Calories

Calories in Sea Food
The calories in fish largely depend on fat content, both visible and invisible. These foods are divided into three groups: lean, moderately fat, and fat. The calorie values below apply to cooked products after visible fat has been removed. Note, when dieting chose only from the lean and moderately fat groups.
Very Lean Shellfish (25 Cal/Oz)
Clams, Crabmeat
Lobster, Mussels
Oysters, Scallops
Shrimp
Lean Fish (50 Cal/Oz)
Abalone, Bluefish
Bonito, Butterfish
Cod, Eels, raw
Flounder, Haddock
Halibut, Herring, raw

Ocean perch
Pike, lake, Pollack
Salmon, fresh or canned
Shad, Shad roe
Sturgeon
Swordfish, Tilefish
Tuna, fresh/canned in water (35 Cal/Oz)
Weakfish, Whitefish
Moderately Fat Fish **(75 Cal/Oz)**
Bass, average
Herring, pickled
Mackerel, Sardines
Trout, brook
Tuna, canned in oil

Calories in Vegetables
Any vegetable may be substituted for any other fruit or vegetable with the same calorie count.
25 Calories per cup
Artichoke (1 medium)
Asparagus (6 spear)
Beans (snap, green, wax)
Cabbage, Cauliflower
Celery, Chard
Cucumber, Endive
Escarole, Lettuce
Mushrooms, Parsley
Peppers, Pickles
Pimentos, Radishes
Scallions
Squash (summer)
Tomato (1 medium)
Tomato juice, Watercress
50 Calories per cup
Bean sprouts, Kohlrabi
Beet greens, Mustard greens
Beets, Broccoli
Brussels sprouts
Carrots, Eggplant

Fennel, Kale
Okra, Rutabagas
Sauerkraut
Spinach
Turnip greens, Turnips
100 Calories per cup
Collards
Dandelion greens
Onion (1 medium)
Parsnips
Potato (1 medium)
Pumpkin, Rice (100 Cal per ½ cup)
Leeks, Squash (winter)
150 Calories per cup
Beans, lima
Corn, Peas
Sweet potato (1 medium)
180 Calories per cup
Tofu

Calories in Fruit

Any fruit may be substituted for any other fruit or vegetable with the same calorie count.
50 Calories per cup (or as indicated)
Apricots (raw, 3)
Cantaloupe (½ medium)
Cranberries, Currants
Fruit salad (raw or water packed)
Gooseberries
Honeydew melon
Lemon or Lime (2 medium)
Lemon or Lime juice
Nectarines (2 small)
Plums (2), Rhubarb
Strawberries
Tangerines (2 small)
Watermelon
75 Calories
Apple (1 medium)

Grapefruit (½ medium)
Orange (1 medium)
100 Cal/cup (or as indicated)
Applesauce, Apricot
Banana (1 medium)
Blackberries
Blueberries
Cherries
Dates (4 raw or dried)
Grapefruit (sections or juice)
Prunes (4 medium)
Figs (3 small), Grapes
Loganberries
Orange (sections or juice)
Papayas
Peaches (raw or canned)
Pears (raw or canned)
Pineapple (raw or juice)
Raspberries
150 Calories per cup
Apple juice, Mango
Grape juice
Persimmons, Guava
Plums (raw or canned)
Prune juice (200 Calories per cup)
Raisins (500 Calories per cup)

Calories in Dairy Products
Whole milk 150 Cal/cup
Skim milk 80 Cal/cup
Yogurt - Whole milk - plain (180 Cal/cup)
Yogurt - Fat-free – plain (90 Cal/cup)
Yogurt – Fat-free - frozen choc (240 Cal/cup)
Cottage cheese - whole milk (220 Cal/cup)
Cottage cheese - fat free (160 Cal/cup)
All other cheese 100 Cal/Oz
Ice cream:
Whole milk (300 Cal/cup)
Light (240 Cal/cup)
Fat free (220 Cal/cup)

Sherbet (250 Cal/cup)
Egg medium (80 Calories)

Bread and Cereals
Bagels (3½" dia) 200 Cal
Biscuits (2" dia) 100.Cal
Cereal Cooked (½ cup)   75 Cal
Cereal Dry (¾ cup) 100 Cal
Corn bread (2" square) 150 Cal
Melba toast (1 piece) 25 Cal
Most bread (1 slice) 65 Cal
Rolls (average) 100 Cal
Ry-Crisp (1 piece) 25 Cal
Crackers, Cookies & Cake
Graham (1 whole cracker) . 100 Cal
Angel food (2 oz) .... 175 Cal

Calories in Oils and Nuts
Butter 50 Calories per pat (16 pats per ¼ lb)
Nuts 100 Calories per handful
Peanut butter 100 Cal/Tbsp
Salad dressings 75 Cal/Tbsp
Vegetable Oils 125 Cal/Tbsp

NoPaperPress eBooks and Paperbacks

100-Day Super Diet-1200 Cal*
100-Day Super Diet-1500 Cal*
100-Day No-Cooking Diet-1200 Cal*
100-Day No-Cooking Diet-1500 Cal*
90-Day Smart Diet-1200 Cal*
90-Day Smart Diet-1500 Cal*
90-Day No-Cooking Diet - 1200 Cal*
90-Day No-Cooking Diet - 1500 Cal*
90-Day Perfect Diet - 1200 Cal*
90-Day Perfect Diet - 1500 Cal*
60-Day Perfect Diet-1200 Cal*
60-Day Perfect Diet-1500 Cal*
50-Day Flex Diet-1200 Cal*
50-Day Flex Diet-1500 Cal*
30-Day Quick Diet - Women*
30-Day Quick Diet for Men*
30-Day No-Cooking Diet*
30-Day Diet - Women - Metric*
30-Day Diet for Men - Metric*
25 Day Easy Diet-1200 Cal*
25 Day Easy Diet-1500 Cal*
25-Day No-Cooking Diet
10-Day Express Diet
10-Day No-Cooking Diet*
7-Day Diet for Women*
7-Day Diet for Men*
7-Day No-Cooking Diets*
90-Day Gluten-Free Diet-1200 Cal*
90-Day Gluten-Free Diet-1500 Cal*
30-Day Gluten-Free Quick Diet*
30-Day Gluten-Free No-Cooking Diet*
7-Day Diet for Women - Metric*
7-Day Diet for Men - Metric
7-Day Gluten-Free Express Diet*
7-Day Gluten-Free No-Cooking Diet*
90-Day Vegetarian Diet-1200 Cal*
90-Day Vegetarian Diet-1500 Cal*
30-Day Vegetarian Diet*
7-Day Vegetarian Diet*
Weight Loss for Women*
Weight Loss for Women - Metric
Weight Loss for Women - UK
Weight Loss for Men*
Maximum Weight Loss - 1200 Cal*
Maximum Weight Loss - 1500 Cal*

Weight Loss for Men - Metric*
Maximum Weight Loss- 1200 Cal*
Maximum Weight Loss- 1500 Cal*
Weight Control - U.S. Edition*
Weight Control - Metric. Edition
Prof Weight Control Women - U.S.
Prof Weight Control Women - Metric
Prof Weight Control Men - U.S.
Prof Weight Control Men - Metric
Weight Maintenance - U.S. Ed*
Weight Maintenance - Metric. Ed*
Weight Maintenance - UK Ed
Weight Loss for Senior Men*
Weight Loss for Senior Women*
Eat Smart - U.S. Edition*
Eat Smart - Metric Edition
30-Day Mediterranean Diet
Exercise Smart - U.S. Edition*
Exercise Smart - Metric Edition
Exercise Smart - UK Edition*
Total Fitness - U.S. Edition
Total Fitness - Metric Edition
Total Fitness - UK Edition
Total Fitness for Women-U.S. Ed*
Total Fitness for Women - Metric
Total Fitness for Women - UK Ed
Total Fitness for Men - U.S. Ed*
Total Fitness for Men- Metric Ed*
Total Fitness for Men - UK Ed
Senior Fitness - U.S. Edition*
Senior Fitness - Metric Edition*
Senior Fitness - UK Edition*
Computer Diet - U.S. Edition*
Computer Diet - Metric Ed*
Reliable Weight Loss - U.S. Ed
101 Weight Loss Tips*
101 Healthy Eating Tips*
101 Lifelong Fitness Tips*
101 Weight Maintenance Tips
101 Weight Loss Recipes
101 GF Weight Loss Recipes
101 Veggie Weight Loss Recipes*
30-Day Mediterranean Diet*
90-Day Mediterranean Diet - 1200 Cal*
90-Day Mediterranean Diet - 1500 Cal*

* These titles are available as both ebooks and paperbacks. Our ebooks are sold by Amazon, Apple, Google, Barnes & Noble and Kobo, but our paperbacks are only sold by Amazon.

Disclaimer

This book offers general meal planning, nutrition and weight control information. It is not a medical manual and the author does not claim to be medically qualified. The material in this book is not intended to be a substitute for medical counseling. Everyone should have a medical checkup before beginning a weight loss program. Moreover, the physician conducting the medical exam should be made aware of and should approve the specific weight control program planned. Additionally, while the author and publisher have made every effort to ensure the accuracy of the information in this book, they make no representations or warranties regarding its accuracy or completeness. Further, neither the author nor publisher assume liability for any medical problems that might result from applying the methods in this book, or for any loss of profit, or any other commercial damages, including but not limited to special, incidental, consequential or other damages, and any such liability is hereby expressly disclaimed.

www.ingramcontent.com/pod-product-compliance
Lightning Source LLC
Chambersburg PA
CBHW060407290526
45791CB00002B/649